Mick Dawson is a professional speaker, sailor, writer and film maker. A former Royal Marine Commando, Mick saw active service in the Falklands War and the Middle East. Following on from his military career Mick pursued his lifelong passion for the Ocean, becoming a professional sailor and ultimately one of the most experienced and successful ocean rowers in the world.

Together with his friend and rowing partner Chris Martin, in 2009 Mick completed the first and still the only successful crossing of the North Pacific in a rowing boat; from Japan to the Iconic Golden Gate Bridge in San Francisco. A voyage of almost 7,000 miles which took Mick and Chris over six months to complete.

Mick has subsequently created the 'Cockleshell Endeavour' project; a resource based on ocean and amphibious challenges designed to assist recovering veterans dealing with physical and mental health issues on their road to recovery.

This book tells the story of the Cockleshell Endeavour.

www.cockleshellendeavour.com

Also by Mick Dawson

Rowing the Pacific: 7,000 Miles from Japan to San Francisco

NEVER LEAVE A MAN BEHIND

Around the Falklands and Rowing across the Pacific

MICK DAWSON

ROBINSON

ROBINSON

First published in Great Britain in 2020 by Robinson

This paperback edition published in 2021 by Robinson

3 5 7 9 10 8 6 4 2

A CIP catalogue record for this book
is available from the British Library.

ISBN: 978-1-47214-403-4

Typeset in Adobe Garamond by Hewer Text UK Ltd, Edinburgh
Printed and bound in Great Britain by Clays Ltd, Elcograf S.p.A.

Papers used by Robinson are from well-managed forests and other responsible sources.

Robinson
An imprint of
Little, Brown Book Group
Carmelite House
50 Victoria Embankment
London EC4Y 0DZ

An Hachette UK Company
www.hachette.co.uk

www.littlebrown.co.uk

I'd like to dedicate this book to two incredible people who, sadly, will never meet. Between them they are responsible for the start of this remarkable story and the successful conclusion to it.

To Jackie Grenham (Mrs G.) and Natalie Harper.
I hope I've done justice to the story you both helped create.

CONTENTS

INTRODUCTION

This book, much like my first, is largely based around waterborne adventures. It appears water may be my natural habitat. The difference with this book, though, is that it's not my story. I'm just a small part of it. It's the story of two men and their battles to overcome major physical and mental health problems unexpectedly forced upon them.

Both former servicemen with very different issues at very different times in their lives, they had one thing in common. The system that was designed to support them when they needed it failed them.

It's not a story of recrimination or bitterness, though, nor is it a story which paints former service personnel as victims or universally damaged. They're not. Quite the opposite. The story of the two Steves in this book is a relentlessly positive one. It shows how combining the physical and mental strengths developed in the service to overcome increasingly formidable challenges enabled them to finally conquer their own problems and disabilities.

I hope their stories will inspire you as much as they inspired me while sharing in their adventures.

CHAPTER 1

HURRICANE LANE

So close.

It was 17 August 2018. After two months at sea and having rowed close to three thousand miles from Monterey Bay in California, we were almost within sight of our destination, Honolulu.

I'm an experienced ocean rower, but my partner, Steve 'Sparky' Sparkes, was not only a complete novice, he is also blind.

If we made it across, Sparky would become the first visually impaired person to row the Pacific. He should get an entry in the Guinness Book of World Records and we'd also raise money for and raise awareness of the continuing plight of UK veterans who've slipped through the support network of every conflict from World War II to the present day. There was a lot riding on our little adventure.

I wrote in the ship's log as a postscript to that day's entry: 'Hurricane Lane has formed well south of us about 360 miles and is currently tracking steadily west.' Tongue in cheek, I finished the entry: 'Is there going to be an unexpected last-minute drama?'

Three days later I'd get the answer. Yes, there was going to be a last-minute drama. A potentially catastrophic one.

Hurricane Lane, which since her birth had mirrored our course west across the Pacific harmlessly, almost four hundred miles south of us, ominously began to slow her progress. At the same time, she was steadily building in ferocity as she fed on the warm waters of the Pacific Ocean beneath her. Ultimately, she grew into a Category 5 storm, the highest classification there is for a hurricane. With wind strengths potentially well in excess of a hundred

1

miles per hour, Lane had now become one of nature's most destructive phenomena and, terrifyingly, she began turning her attention towards us.

Unusually for hurricanes forming in that part of the Pacific, she changed course unexpectedly, twice, steadily arcing her path north, towards the Hawaiian Islands. And us. By 21 August, Hawaii was bracing itself for only the second Category 5 hurricane in history to strike its shores.

Sparky and I, on our intrepid rowing boat *Bojangles*, were bracing ourselves for our first.

Initially I'd decided not to tell Sparky about Lane until it became clear whether the storm would affect us or not. I knew hurricanes seldom make landfall in the Hawaiian Islands, so there seemed at that time no major cause for concern. Sparky was in severe pain from a compression fracture to his shoulder, which had all but crippled him for several weeks. Exhausted from over two months at sea, battling endless challenges, now constantly in pain, he really didn't need anything else to worry about.

The day before Lane turned her attention towards us, I'd received a weather report from the race organisers saying the storm was forecast to continue heading west, staying well south of our position until eventually decaying and dying deep in the Pacific, hundreds of miles west of Hawaii. It was unlikely we'd suffer any noticeable affects from the storm's passage as we completed our final few miles into Honolulu. It was the news I'd hoped for and expected to hear, but I was still relieved and told Sparky right away.

'Mate,' I said cheerfully, 'just to let you know, we've had a hurricane forming south-east of us over the last few days. Hurricane Lane. I didn't want to say anything about it until I knew if it would affect us or not. Happy to say the latest weather forecast has it passing south of us heading due west in the next day or so and shouldn't bother us at all.'

'Thank God for that,' he answered sombrely. 'I think we've had enough to deal with without getting run down by a bloody hurricane as well.'

It was welcome good news and it lifted morale for both of us as we looked at last towards the final two or three days on board and what increasingly appeared to be our imminent successful arrival in Honolulu.

The following day I stared in disbelief at the new weather forecast in front of me. It was from my old rowing partner and friend Chris Martin, the race organiser and director. He had been so inspired by our voyage in 2009 across the North Pacific, from Japan to San Francisco, that he'd gone on to set up the now biannual Great Pacific Race, from Monterey Bay in California to Honolulu. We were taking part in its third incarnation.

The news was bad, and he obviously wanted to be the one to let me know. It seemed Lane had changed direction and was now on a collision course with the Hawaiian Islands, and by virtue of that heading straight for us, a hundred miles offshore, heading towards Honolulu in a seven-metre-long ocean rowing boat.

In addition to being bad luck, it was also potentially life-threatening. Somewhere deep in my subconscious, even as, incredulously, I read the forecast, I wasn't surprised. It was almost as if I'd known, from Lane's initial inception just a few days earlier, that she was going to impact our arrival. During our voyage we'd christened the trip 'The death of a thousand cuts', because of the endless unexpected hurdles we'd had to overcome. The question now was: would this be the final cut?

Despite that, and not for the first time in my ocean rowing career, I read and reread the weather forecast in front of me, willing the information contained in it to miraculously change to a more helpful prognosis. It didn't. The forecast was what it was. No matter how many times I read it, the news didn't get any better, but waiting for divine intervention to strike at least gave me time to let the reality settle in.

I recognised the situation and, more importantly, what options were available to us. One: stay on board, batten down the hatches and attempt to ride the hurricane out. Two: row as fast as we could and desperately try to make landfall in Honolulu ahead of the storm. Or three: call for rescue and get off the boat before the potentially deadly storm hit.

After more than two months at sea, overcoming what seemed like an endless stream of increasingly devastating and demoralising challenges and with success almost within our grasp, it appeared the cruellest outcome of all awaited us: ignominious failure just in sight of the finish line.

I called Chris on the satellite phone to discuss the options, and to hopefully discover at least some small measure of positive news. I was pleasantly surprised to discover there was some. The projected path of the storm meant if we deployed the parachute anchor to halt our progress, we would be in the safest possible position to survive the storm. (The parachute anchor is exactly that – a parachute dropped into the water on the end of 250 feet of line attached to the stern of the boat. It inflates beneath the surface of the water as a normal parachute inflates in the air and then acts as a giant drogue in the ocean. It slows the boat and prevents it from going backwards too swiftly in adverse winds, but more importantly it helps prevent the boat capsizing in a storm.) Deploying the parachute anchor at our present location would slow our progress west, if not halt it, but keep us in a position where we could escape the worst of the hurricane's ferocious winds.

We were in the survivable quadrant of the hurricane, so our luck hadn't deserted us completely. The bad news was that every mile further west we progressed would bring increasingly powerful wind speeds and the mountainous seas those winds would generate.

With Lane's progress across the Pacific once again picking up pace, racing the storm into Honolulu would almost certainly see us caught just offshore when she hit. That would be a deadly situation for any vessel, let alone a small ocean rowing boat. Chris suggested optimistically that there was the possibility of running for the sanctuary of a slightly closer port on a nearer island. Even that option left us vulnerable to being caught at sea just as the storm arrived.

There were then two viable options. Stay on the boat and try to ride out the hurricane that was barrelling towards us or call for help and get off as soon as possible.

My natural inclination was to stay and ride the storm out. I'd built *Bo* to survive exactly the conditions which were coming, and I was confident she would keep us safe as she always had done on the six-month crossing of the North Pacific Chris Martin and I had completed nine years earlier. Severe weather was a constant issue on that voyage of almost seven thousand miles and *Bo* had carried us safely through everything that the North Pacific had thrown at us.

But Sparky was injured, constantly in considerable pain and discomfort from his damaged shoulder, and exhausted. The sole purpose of our voyage, which we'd named The Cockleshell Pacific Endeavour, was for him to become the first visually impaired person to row the Pacific Ocean. We wanted to show the world that blindness didn't have to limit what you could achieve. One thing was for certain, though, whichever course of action we followed, it was Sparky's decision.

'Mate, you know that hurricane I mentioned yesterday?'

'The one that's "going to miss us"?' He emphasised going to miss us almost as if it was a promise which I was about to break.

'Yeah. That one. Well,' – I paused, before breaking that unspoken promise – 'I've just had an update. It's changed direction and it's not going to miss us now. In fact, it's heading straight for us. And just for good measure it's been upgraded to Category 5.' Sparky may have lost his sight, but he was a former Royal Marine. He could deal with the facts however harsh. He would insist on them.

There was a pause. Sparky was out on deck near the front hatch, wrapped in his foul-weather jacket. Despite the proximity to Hawaii, it was still a cold day with frequent squally showers. He didn't react immediately as he allowed the news to sink in.

Finally, he said quietly, 'Seriously? You're not taking the piss, are you?'

'No mate. I'm not taking the piss.'

'For f—' He didn't finish the word or his sentence. He didn't need to. I could hear the anguish and frustration in his voice. Two, maybe three, days from finishing and now this. It would have broken many people.

'We've basically got two choices,' I said to him. 'We put the para anchor in now and get ready to ride it out. Or we call for rescue and get off the boat before the storm hits. The good news is we're in the best position to ride the storm out and in the best boat. We can survive this, mate. *Bo*'s built to do just that. But make no mistake, this is a life-threatening situation and there are no guarantees. It must be your call. Whichever decision you make, I'll happily go along with it,' I lied. I would never have happily left *Bo*.

I paused for a few seconds before asking solemnly, 'Well? Do you want to get off, mate?'

He turned towards me and said slowly, 'Of course I fucking want to get off!' My heart sank. He paused for a few seconds longer, staring into the distance before carrying on. 'But I'm not going to, am I? Do you think I've come all this way to let you and everybody else down now? We'll stay on board and ride the bastard out!'

He slowly turned towards me, a typically broad grin spreading across his face.

'Anyway,' he said. 'I've been through a hurricane before.'

'Really?' I replied doubtfully. 'When?'

'When I was in the corps in 1984 on HMS *Hermes*. In the middle of the Atlantic, no big deal,' he said dismissively.

I smiled and shook my head. 'Mate. HMS *Hermes* was an aircraft carrier . . . We're on a rowing boat. This is going to be a bit different.'

He shrugged his shoulders and smiled. 'Right,' he said, 'what do we need to do first?'

Decision made. We began to prepare *Bo* and ourselves for the deadly storm, all the time trying not to think too deeply about what the next couple of days might have in store for us.

The days that followed would indeed prove to be among the most terrifying and challenging of our Cockleshell Endeavour experiences. But they weren't the start of them. The Pacific row had, in effect, been born on the top of a windswept Falkland Islands mountain overlooking Port Stanley four years earlier . . .

CHAPTER 2

THE BIRTH OF THE COCKLESHELL ENDEAVOUR

The phone call came as a surprise. The request that came with it, an even greater one.

It was Tony Grenham, the brother of a good friend of mine, Steve Grenham. Steve, a fellow former Royal Marine, who lived in Brighton, my neck of the woods whenever I'm back in England. On more than one occasion over the years, Steve and I, occasionally together with Tony, had emerged from the local pubs somewhat worse for wear after a few too many beers and a night of reminiscing and putting the world to rights. I considered them good friends, with Steve one of my closest.

'Mick? Could you arrange for a flight for Steve to go back to the Falkland Islands for me, mate?' Tony asked out of the blue. 'Apparently, as a veteran he's intitled to subsidised flights to go back. Mum wants to sort it for his fiftieth birthday. She thinks he needs it, that it'll do him good.'

Steve, like me, was a veteran of the 1982 Falklands War, when Argentina briefly occupied the far-flung British dependency located in the South Atlantic. As young marines we were both part of the task force that sailed from the UK to liberate the islands.

The suggestion Steve required any 'doing good' came as a shock. I had no idea that he had any issues relating to his experiences during the conflict. The signs were undoubtedly there, I know now, but I simply hadn't picked up on them.

I soon discovered that flights to and from the islands were indeed available, provided by the Ministry of Defence. They came at a heavily reduced rate on board the Royal Air Force flights supplying the islands. The RAF air bridge, as it was called, offered a limited number of seats on its weekly flights, subject to operational demands, for veterans of the conflict. Steve was most certainly entitled to one.

I gave Steve's mum the good news. Mrs G. was a lovely, flame-haired, no-nonsense lady, down-to-earth and with a wickedly dry sense of humour. Although troubled with ill health, I knew her as a constantly upbeat and positive lady, great fun and great company. In many ways she reminded me of my own mum. They each had one defining quality: they lived for their two sons.

Sadly, Steve's dad had passed away long before I had a chance to meet him, but in his absence Mrs G. was the rock at the centre of the tight-knit family. If Mrs G. was worried about Steve, there would be good reason. With that in mind I was more than happy to be able to play a part in creating something she felt would help her son.

'Why don't you go with him?' she said to me a few days later, when I rang to confirm Steve's seat was booked.

I was oddly shocked at the suggestion and a little lost for words. I'd never thought about returning to the islands. It was a major part of my life but a distant memory now. It had simply never occurred to me to go back. Why would I want to?

'He'd enjoy it more if he was going with somebody he knew,' Mrs G. encouraged. 'Why not go? You both earned it.'

The more I thought about it, the more it seemed not only a good idea but also a once-in-a-lifetime opportunity. Why not? It was an affordable chance to visit one of the most remote and fascinating places on earth, and this time nobody would be trying to kill me. I decided to take Mrs G.'s advice and booked myself a seat along with Steve.

Decision made, I began to look forward to what I hoped would be a unique and enjoyable experience. It would prove to be both. I had no idea at that point, though, that very much like my first visit to the Falkland Islands, it would also become a life-changing one.

CHAPTER 3

THE RETURN

Our return to the Falkland Islands began on a cold, dark December morning in 2014, early enough to leave the roads clear of traffic and the pair of us bleary eyed and yawning. It was going to be a long day. Steve's brother Tony had generously given up the comfort of his own bed to drive us to the base we were due to fly from in Oxfordshire: RAF Brize Norton.

A modern military system, noticeably more civilised and welcoming than either of us remembered from our time in the service, saw us swiftly, politely and efficiently processed and awaiting our flight to the southern hemisphere. Little more than nine hours later we found ourselves disembarking at the only scheduled stop on our journey south, Ascension Island.

Ascension is an isolated volcanic island nestling centrally in the Atlantic Ocean, just south of the equator, almost midway between Africa and Brazil. It provides a natural stop-off point for any journey between Great Britain and the Falklands whether by sea or air. It has a population of less than a thousand people, none of whom are indigenous to the island. A tiny relic of what remains of the British Empire, its role is to provide bases for the American and British military and, now that we're in more modern times, a monitoring station for the European Space Agency. In 1982, Ascension was the last chance to take on supplies and reposition men and equipment for the forthcoming landings.

I remember when the task force set off from the UK there was a surreal atmosphere. Ships and units hurriedly prepared for a war at the other end of the world in a matter of days. Dozens of ships;

thousands of men. It was an incredible logistical achievement, even before a single vessel slipped her moorings and headed south. The fact that the majority of Royal Marine commandos and para-troopers, who would go on to do the bulk of the fighting on land, were billeted on the requisitioned luxury cruise liner SS *Canberra* only added to that sense of unreality – fuelling, at least initially, a carnival-like atmosphere.

Before the Argentine invasion few people in the British Isles had even heard of the Falkland Islands. Of those who had, many thought they were located somewhere off Scotland. Now the biggest British military force to go into action since World War II was steaming eight thousand miles south to liberate British subjects from a modern, well-equipped, well-trained and, with every passing day, increasingly well-prepared occupying army.

It seemed inconceivable, despite the Argentine invasion, that this conflict would escalate further. There was no real history of animosity between Argentina and Britain despite the South American nation's loudly voiced and long held, if tenuous, claim to the islands. Surely the politicians on both sides would eventually see sense and negotiate a peaceful solution?

But by the time the task force arrived in Ascension it was becoming very clear the politicians were not going to find that solution. Even if they wanted to, rhetoric was becoming increasingly confrontational and negotiations fruitless. Full-blown conflict, it seemed, was unavoidable. The upbeat party mood that pervaded the first part of our voyage south began to dissipate. As we reached Ascension few of us were in any doubt that we were now preparing for war.

Thirty-two years later, as Steve and I emerged from the grey fuselage of our Royal Air Force transport plane, we were hit with the brutal impact of the island's desert heat. We made our way down the disembarkation steps and, along with our fellow passengers, were ushered to an enclosed outdoor area close to the runway apron. It was an extension of a small building that apparently served as the airport terminal. The secure compound area along with an indoor lounge and cafe provided us with a place to sit and relax while our aircraft was refuelled for the final part of our journey south. A welcome cup of tea and a less welcome sandwich of indeterminate identity helped us pass the time. As we sat chatting, for the first time it finally began to sink in that we were returning, after all these years, to the Falkland Islands.

The flight from the UK had been comfortable and pleasant. Probably as a direct result of that, nothing up until that point had reminded us of our original journey. The slick departure process in 2014 bore no similarity to the urgent, rapid and at times chaotic ship embarkations that were the hallmark of our original trip. A comfortable flight on a modern aircraft, over in a few hours, bore no resemblance to the days and weeks on board ship battling through the often-mountainous seas of the Atlantic Ocean, slowly and anxiously making our way towards our distant destination and the confrontation that awaited.

Now, though, having stepped off the plane, we were greeted by a familiar landscape and a climate which looked and felt exactly as it had all those years previously. Memories and stories slowly came back. Ascension was exactly as we remembered it, harsh and unforgiving, a rocky oasis, providing an incongruous final landfall before the Falkland Islands and the experiences that lay ahead of us.

One particular memory from that brief stop at Ascension in 1982 has remained with me. We were watching one of the three fighting companies (about a hundred marines) from 45 Commando attempting to embark on a landing craft in a fierce Atlantic swell. My troop had just finished a speed march, a timed run with full kit and weapons – making the most of the brief time on dry land to break up the monotony and limitations of the endless circuit training on board ship. Exhausted and sweating after our efforts, we'd gathered to watch the spectacle developing on the beach.

The waves were crashing violently onto the exposed shore. The large landing craft utility, or LCU, was at the mercy of those ferocious waves, as were the marines. With the ramp at the front of the craft lowered to allow the troops to board, the LCU – which was big enough to transport a battle tank – was being driven ramp first onto the beach. Due to the ferocious nature of the waves it was regularly being picked up and hurled violently forwards ten or fifteen feet further onto the beach, despite the best efforts of the coxswain driving the vessel to prevent this. Embarkation for our fellow marines was proving perilous, as they attempted to time their run onto the landing craft between those violent surges. Any semblance of an organised embarkation drill was long abandoned and it was now a case of every man for himself.

For the guys involved it must have been a nightmare. For us it provided, with typical British military black humour, an amusing break from our own particular challenges. We joined in from the comfort of the rocks overlooking the beach with good-natured jeers and cheers as one after another of our fellow marines waded into the surf, preparing to time their run and make a leap of faith onto the precarious ramp.

Then, alarmingly, in the middle of all this chaos, one guy stalled his run just at the critical point where he should have leapt on board. He was a distinctive character – tall, powerfully built, with tight curly blond hair. He stood out even before he mistimed his effort to board. His delay left him static in the surf, having lost all momentum. As he attempted to save the situation, leaping forwards with one leg outstretched, the landing craft lurched forwards once more on another breaking wave. The huge ramp scooped him up, one leg either side, crashing down onto the beach with him pinned beneath it. Our cheering ended – the atmosphere had changed in a moment. It was a violent impact. If he wasn't dead, the marine had to be seriously injured. Black humour evaporated and we watched anxiously as the remainder of his comrades on the beach raced to help him, while the coxswain of the landing craft desperately and loudly threw his engines into reverse.

Little more than the marine's distinctive blond hair and the top of his shoulders remained above the tumbling surf. Of his lower body, only his leading leg still hooked around the top of the ramp was still visible, the rest of his presumably broken body was trapped beneath it. We all anticipated the worst, but, incredibly, even before his comrades were able to reach him, he managed to drag himself free. He clambered to his feet before finally, groggily, he turned and leapt onto the now relatively stationary landing craft. Injured pride aside, he seemed completely unhurt. A broad grin spread across his face as he turned towards his now mightily relieved audience from the safety of the landing craft deck. A fist punch into the air signalling his success, or perhaps just his relief at the outcome. Either way, it was greeted with huge cheers from those of us assembled on and around the beach.

It was a quite remarkable escape. I can only assume the breaking seas must have churned up the sand and reduced the solidity of the beach where the ramp came down, preventing him being crushed between it and the surface of the beach. He must have had just enough time to wrestle himself free before the weight of the vessel fully bore down, crushing him.

That memory has always stayed with me, but its significance only became clear many years later. That incident, in equal measures funny and terrifying, was the first and most vivid glimpse I would have of the arbitrary nature of luck, and even more importantly luck's huge significance in the shaping of all our lives. As we'd all soon discover in the conflict to come, many lives would be changed in many ways purely due to the vagaries of luck. The nature of that change hinged on whether your luck was good or bad.

Regardless of the level of your abilities and despite the most thorough preparation, luck could and often would prove to be the crucial factor between success and failure, or even life and death, in our war, as it had been in previous wars and as it has continued to be in subsequent conflicts. For everyone involved in the Falklands War, luck would become our most precious commodity.

It's a truth that applies equally to everyday life, but one that we can easily overlook as we get on with the seemingly all-consuming day-to-day activities of our normal existence. The intense, pressure-cooker atmosphere of war, however, allows for a far greater and more singular focus on the nature of luck and how your fate can be governed by it.

A few years later, as I was preparing to leave the Royal Marines, I found myself serving in the same establishment as the blond-haired marine who'd had such a lucky escape. By then he was a corporal. His name was Gary 'Gaz' Marshall, still as distinguishable by virtue of his build and his hair as he had been that day on the beach on Ascension.

In the fighting that followed to liberate the Falklands, Gaz was awarded the Military Medal for his distinguished actions on patrol around Two Sisters, one of the strategically important mountains surrounding Port Stanley. The Military Medal is the second highest award in the British military for acts of outstanding bravery in the face of the enemy, the Victoria Cross being the highest. His ability to board a landing craft in rough seas obviously was no reflection on his ability as a soldier or his incredible level of courage.

It hasn't been lost on me that without that stroke of luck that saved him on the beach as he stumbled beneath the crushing weight of that landing craft, none of his subsequent actions would have happened. How many other lives would have been affected in how many different ways without that one random stroke of luck on a remote beach in the middle of the Atlantic Ocean? What could have been a life-changing, if not life-ending, accident, by virtue of luck, transformed a potentially terminal situation into little more than an amusing story of a lucky escape on the way to a much more important adventure.

All our lives hang daily on that tightrope between disaster and success if we analyse them closely enough. We seldom do. That's probably why we are so often found guilty of taking so much for granted. Perhaps if we did look at life more closely – how unique it is, how fragile and fleeting, and how quickly it can change – we would have a totally different attitude as to how we choose to live it.

That creeping realisation for me, that life is so brief and precious, became the driving force behind how I've lived my life since the Falklands War and why I've made my decisions and choices, right and wrong. Life has to be lived to the full and, above all, it has to have meaning. It has to matter. We're all going to die; we have no choice in that. The choice comes in how we live, what we do, and what we try to achieve while we're here.

Oddly enough, that story had far greater significance for me, merely a spectator of events, than it ever did for Gaz. When I reminded him of it probably no more than six years later, he smiled and almost dismissed it. To him it was a barely remembered near miss.

'A bit of a nightmare,' he laughed, 'but no big deal.'

He was lucky. It was just a very small part of the far bigger, far more significant story that would follow for him and for all of us.

For me, the incident on the beach was the start of my realisation, if only on a subconscious level, that life is governed to some extent by fate. I believe your destiny or, as I prefer to think of it, your potential, is largely set, at least in terms of direction. Luck is the tool fate brings into play when we are heading off the path we're meant to be on. Luck, good or bad, is fate's way of trying to guide you back to the path you are destined to pursue, the path that your unique strengths and passions give you, if you allow them, the best tools to follow.

Of course, I may choose to have that view or belief because I consider myself to have been very fortunate. The luck that has governed my life consistently has almost always been good. It certainly proved to be good during my experiences in the Falklands War in 1982, and many times since, not least during my ocean rowing adventures. I've had cause to thank many times the lucky stars that seem to shine over my life. The story contained in my first book, *Rowing the Pacific*, bears witness to that, and I believe the story in this book echoes those sentiments. One thing is for certain, after my adventures during the Falklands War in 1982, nobody could ever accuse me of taking life for granted.

With our focus steadily turning towards our return to the islands, Steve and I reboarded our now fully fuelled aircraft and prepared for take-off on the last leg of our journey south. With the stop in Ascension and with each passing hour we were both increasingly growing into the journey neither of us had been 100 per cent convinced of when we set off. The decision to return was beginning to feel like a good decision, the right decision, for both of us.

Flying south towards the bottom of the world for another eight hours, with nothing but the Atlantic Ocean beneath us, we

greeted with weary relief the pilot's announcement of our imminent arrival at RAF Mount Pleasant, the Falklands' sole military
airport. Steadily the aircraft began to shed its cruising altitude,
eventually dropping into bumpy, ominously dark clouds. Just a
few hundred feet above East Falkland, we finally broke through
the base layer of those turbulent rain-soaked clouds that had been
masking our view. There beneath us, at last, stretching haphaz-
ardly in all directions out into the hostile Southern Ocean, we saw
the Falkland Islands for the first time in more than thirty years.
The unique, bleak, harsh, wind-sculpted rock-and-peat landscape
was immediately familiar.

Those dark clouds we'd so recently emerged from were dump-
ing torrential levels of rain into the driving westerly wind that
welcomed us as we stepped off the aircraft. It was freezing, windy
and wet, exactly as we remembered it. We were back.

CHAPTER 4

HELP!

The grim weather which greeted us on our arrival in no way reflected the warm welcome we were to receive everywhere and from everyone during our stay on the islands. Our base for the visit was Liberty Lodge in Port Stanley. Self-catering accommodation built specifically for returning veterans, it's immaculately kept by the Falklands Veterans Association and very comfortable. It stands as a glowing testament to the ongoing gratitude, warmth and hospitality of the Falkland Islanders to the troops who once came to their aid. Steve and I had our own room and I was gleefully informed by the lady who greeted us that Prince Harry had been the last person to sleep in my bed prior to an expedition to the South Pole. We only had four short days before our flight home so we planned to spend that time visiting as many of the places we could that were significant to us both from our experiences in 1982. The first thing we did, much to the surprise of our hosts in Liberty Lodge, was go swimming. I'd worked out on the flight down that I'd swum in the middle of every ocean on the planet, except for the Southern Ocean – this would be my only opportunity to put that right. Steve was up for it, so, early on our first morning, Gary Clement drove us, with two disbelieving ex-Matelots (Royal Navy sailors) along to spectate, to the appropriately named Surf Bay. 'This is a first,' Gary informed us dryly, as we leapt into the tumbling, freezing waves of the Southern Ocean.

On our last full day on the islands, Steve and I found ourselves steadily ascending Mount Harriet on the outskirts of Port Stanley. Harriet is one of a range of low-lying mountains that surround and dominate the island's capital. Little more than 250 metres high, Harriet and her sisters emerge from the bleak and flat Falkland Island landscape like angry, rocky scars. Mountains only by virtue of their Falkland Island setting, they were still of huge tactical significance militarily. After the landings and as the fighting progressed, they became the scene for the final and decisive actions in the war. Marines, paratroopers and the Scots Guards who'd arrived with the second wave of British troops fought a series of formidable and vicious battles at night on their slopes. We ultimately won them all, forcing the Argentine forces to retreat in desperation back to Stanley, their final refuge before their inevitable surrender, which came on 14 June.

Harriet was where Steve fought in 1982, as an eighteen-year-old marine with 42 Commando in J Company, as part of a diversionary attack on the eastern flank. At the top of the mountain in December 2014, having described to me in straightforward but vivid detail that grim night's battle he'd fought in three decades previously, Steve stopped and turned to me. He explained that at the insistence of his wife, Aicha, and his family, he'd recently approached one of the principal military charities in the UK for help.

They all felt he was having problems with his mental health and were increasingly worried about his well-being. Typically, Steve didn't consider he had any issues at all and thought they were overreacting. They, however, had seen the steady change in his personality and behaviour over the years and were desperate for him to seek help. The charity unofficially acknowledged he was almost certainly suffering from PTSD after his first informal appointment. Apparently he ticked all the boxes apart from suicidal inclination.

To my astonishment, Steve told me that the charity had then advised him to 'go away. No drugs or alcohol for three months, then come back and we'll diagnose you officially.'

His exact words to me were, 'If I could do that, Mick, I wouldn't need their help, would I?'

On the top of Mount Harriet, next to the simple but powerful white cross which stands as a memorial to those men who lost their lives that night, I saw a friend at his lowest point. Having finally asked for help, the door had been firmly shut in his face. He was isolated and abandoned by the very system that was set up to support him.

I knew something had to be done. Asking for help would not have come easy to Steve. I could tell by his manner he was angry and resented the charity for their response, although inside I'm sure it only reinforced his belief that he didn't really need help. Their response offered no achievable way forwards for Steve and served only to create an immediate and unconquerable barrier between him and the very organisation that was put in place to support him. One thing I knew for certain: Steve would never ask for their help again. This was a critical time for him – a fork in the road at a junction he might never find again. I had to find a way to help.

I considered his words for a few seconds, letting their significance sink in.

'How about we create a project to get you through those three months, mate?' I suggested.

'What kind of project?' he asked.

I hadn't thought of that. I looked around from the top of the mountain at the rugged island coastline stretching out in all directions in the ferocious Southern Ocean surrounding us. I thought for a minute longer, then said: 'I know! We can kayak around the Falklands. How hard can that be?'

Very hard, as it happens. In fact, in terms of kayaking ambitions, it's one of the most challenging you could come up with. Looking back now, I realise it might have saved a considerable amount of hard work and not a small amount of expense if I'd come up with that idea standing on the Isle of Wight rather than the Falkland Islands.

Nonetheless, at that moment, on the summit of Mount Harriet, overlooking Port Stanley, the idea was born. We would create a project to paddle around the Falkland Islands. It would help get Steve back on track and get him in a position to receive the help he needed from the charity set up to look after people in his situation.

Now we needed a name for our adventure.

CHAPTER 5

THE COCKLESHELL HEROES

My previous North Pacific rowing projects had all been under the banner of The Golden Gate Endeavour, a name which I felt highlighted both the ultimate goal, the Golden Gate Bridge, together with the challenging but by no means certain nature of the undertaking, summed up by the word endeavour. We were going to try, but there was no guarantee. Any challenge which guarantees success simply isn't a challenge.

Our Falkland Islands kayaking ambitions were going to be as difficult as my previous ocean rowing adventures, so continuing the 'endeavour' link was a natural choice for the title. The Cockleshell bit came from our shared Royal Marine heritage.

The Cockleshell Heroes was the name of a 1955 film that immortalised an intrepid band of Royal Marines who, during World War II, undertook a daring commando raid on German shipping moored in the port of Bordeaux. Led by Major 'Blondie' Hasler, they paddled two-man canoes along the Gironde Estuary and into the port of Bordeaux. Dropped by the submarine HMS *Tuna* off the French coast, in December 1942 they entered and paddled up the Gironde under cover of darkness, lying low during daylight hours to avoid detection, before placing magnetic limpet mines beneath the waterline to sink the German cargo ships moored in the port. The sturdy canvas canoes used on the raid (codenamed 'Cockles') gave the raiding party their name: The Cockleshell Heroes.

Of the ten marines who took part in the raid, two died from hypothermia after capsizing while navigating the treacherous tidal flow of the Gironde at the entrance. Six of the remaining commandos were eventually captured. Unforgivably they were then murdered by the Nazis as a result of Hitler's infamous 'commando order', which directed that all captured commandos were to be executed, not treated as prisoners of war.

Two managed to escape: Major 'Blondie' Hasler, the architect and commanding officer of the raid, and his paddling partner Corporal Bill Sparks (no relation to Steve Sparkes). Scuttling their kayak, with the help of the French resistance they completed a perilous overland journey to freedom across the Pyrenees mountains to Spain and on to their eventual repatriation to Great Britain, via Gibraltar.

Neither Steve Grenham nor I would suggest for one second that we were carved from the same granite rock as those remarkable men. But we were both a product of the same unique Royal Marine family that has continued to grow from their example, and many others. Our project, in its own way, would also have to be built on the same confident, against-all-odds optimism. We'd accepted a difficult challenge, set a formidable goal, but we were confident we could deliver against the odds, much like them. We liked to think that they would have recognised the spirit and the ambition of what we were trying to achieve. Most importantly, when we were successful, it would provide a fitting tribute to their memory and their continuing inspiration.

All we had to do now was learn to kayak.

CHAPTER 6

NO SUCH THING AS COINCIDENCE

If over the years my steadily increasing belief that fate plays a huge part in life needed any reinforcement, the circumstances of how I met Steve Grenham, and later Sparky, certainly brought that.

In 1997 I found myself living, temporarily, in Brighton on the south coast of England. I'd finished one sailing job and was waiting for the start date of the next contract abroad. I wanted some time at home, and Brighton seemed like a good place to go. It would prove to be the beginning of my love affair with the south coast town; a wonderful, vibrant and bustling place full of creativity, diversity and, most importantly, at least for me, situated by the sea.

It was the day of a big England *v.* France rugby match and I wanted to find a bar that was showing the game. I found myself wandering along a main street I'd never explored before on the outskirts of the city. I passed plenty of pubs but none were showing the match. I thought I was going to be out of luck when, by chance, I came to a junction in the road and looked down a gentle slope to my left. In the distance there appeared to be a small corner pub tucked away almost out of sight. As I approached, much to my delight and relief, I could see inside TV screens showing the immediate build up to the England–France rugby match. A miracle. I was saved!

The pub was called The Wellington. I'd never seen it before, had never even heard of it, and it would take a while and require some effort before I ever found it again. But that afternoon The Wellington turned out to be an incredibly fortunate if unexpected discovery. Not only did it provide a venue to watch a rugby match, it was the catalyst for a whole series of future adventures.

Inside there was a mixture of good-natured locals and rugby fans, hosted by a friendly and welcoming landlord. It was a proper pub, not a soulless chain, and the perfect place to watch a game of rugby. I didn't know anyone, so I found a spot at the bar, out of the way but with a good view of the TV and, equally importantly, easy access for a resupply of Guinness. I remember little of significance now about the game other than it finished with a close, hard-fought victory to the French, which put an end to England's championship dreams for yet another year.

What I do remember is the sound of a faintly familiar voice somewhere behind me that suddenly grabbed my attention. I turned to see if it was someone I knew, unlikely as that was. In the throng surrounding me I couldn't put any specific face to the voice I thought I'd heard. The voice itself was instantly swallowed by the rumbling background din of everyone else's animated conversation. I must have been imagining it, I thought, and returned my attention to the rugby.

Later that afternoon, as the final whistle sounded, I made to leave. Draining the remnants of beer from my pint glass, I placed it on the bar, thanked the landlord for his hospitality and turned to go. At precisely the same time, Steve Grenham, who I would discover had been standing just a few yards along the packed bar all afternoon, did exactly the same. We literally walked into each other.

'Mickey Dawson!' he said, incredulous.

'Steve Grenham!' I said, equally taken aback. The half-familiar voice I'd heard earlier now made sense.

'Well,' he said laughing, 'looks like I won't be going home after all then! Pint?'

*　　*　　*

We drifted into a long and drunken night on a sea of shared memories and half-forgotten stories which reignited a friendship that had begun when we served in the same troop together after the Falklands War. We hadn't seen or heard from each other in over a decade.

I have many great friends from my time in the marines and, regardless of how many years pass between meeting any of them, one thing is universal: it feels like it was yesterday when we do. That's the nature and depth of those friendships. Meeting Steve again was no different; within seconds it seemed like yesterday. There was, however, one thing that was different about Steve from pretty much everyone else I'd known in the corps.

In 1986, when we were serving together, we'd travelled up to the north of England with our troop for 'adventure training'. We were in Fleetwood, just outside the famous seaside resort of Blackpool on England's west coast. On a night out I had a very poignant conversation with Steve, one I've never forgotten. It was the first time he'd spoken in any detail about his experiences in the Falklands with me and probably the first time he'd spoken about one specific event with anyone. It was apparent even then that the experience had stayed with him and had had a lingering impact.

It had been towards the end of the assault on Mount Harriet, he explained. The slopes of the mountain were still shrouded in darkness, the battle all but won but not yet over. An Argentine soldier, evidently cut off from his comrades, had popped up in the distance, out of cover.

Armed and still in the midst of battle, Steve said the whole of his company had instantly opened fire on the figure who'd promptly gone to ground, presumably hit. A few seconds later, the figure popped up again only to be met with another ferocious volley of gunfire. Remarkably the Argentine soldier, instead of trying to surrender, rose from cover and again made another desperate dash to safety, only to be met with another ferocious barrage of fire. This bizarre game of cat and mouse carried on until the soldier darted from cover one final time and the game, along with his life, came to an end.

'He didn't get up from that one,' Steve finished. There was nothing triumphant or disrespectful about Steve's recollection of events, just a resigned recognition.

It was a sad but not unusual story of the violence and brutality of battle, and I'm not proud to admit my reaction at the time was to simply shrug and almost laugh off the farcical circumstances of the unfortunate Argentine's death.

'Do you know what I remember most about that, Mick?' he asked, before pausing and then answering his own question. 'By the end we were all laughing like lunatics. Here was this poor fucker, somebody's son or brother, fighting for his life and we were laughing like lunatics trying to kill him. A few weeks earlier we were on a cruise ship without a care in the world and there we were less than three weeks later, like a bunch of fucking psychopaths, laughing our tits off at somebody dying.' He paused, seemingly considering his words. 'Scary what it can do to you, isn't it?' he said matter-of-factly, before returning to the drink he was holding.

I've never forgotten that conversation, and over the years I've shared it with many people, its significance slowly dawning on me: few veterans from the Falklands, myself included, would have dwelled on that incident in the way which Steve had.

Many years later, as I write this book, most if not all of my friends who fought in 1982 have a more mellow and compassionate view regarding their experiences and their attitude towards our enemies. Some have even built friendships with our former foes. In 1986, when Steve and I had that chat, that compassionate attitude simply didn't exist. Argentinian troops remained the enemy. In the immediate aftermath we were still in the mindset you have to be in to cope with that sort of brutal and unforgiving experience: dismissive and detached from events and, most importantly, detached from the fact that the people you fought and who were killed were human beings. All our empathy lay with our lost comrades. Even in death we were on different sides.

This lack of empathy, a sort of detachment, is true in all wars. Perhaps it's simply a natural coping mechanism that allows people to deal with the undoubted shock and trauma of battle. In Steve however, empathy was his first reaction to those events and probably speaks volumes for his character.

I'm not a psychiatrist so can claim no medical expertise on this, but I believe Steve's future battles with the effects of PTSD date back to his experiences on Mount Harriet. The slow but steady change in his personality in the years that followed was the first indication, had anyone realised, that he was having problems dealing with those experiences.

If it happened now, I'm pleased to say, there is a comprehensive support system in place to respond immediately and provide support. It's by no means a perfect system; it's still evolving, and there can never be any room for complacency. The Royal Marines have been at the vanguard of developing and creating key elements of that support system, implementing a process called TRIM (trauma risk management), which is designed to address potential issues immediately after any traumatic incident.

In the 1980s, when PTSD was not officially recognised as a condition, those suffering with the symptoms were often misdiagnosed, labelled as malingerers or even ridiculed. The only solution at hand was a simple one: go to the pub. Most guys did. Some never came out again.

When Steve's problems first emerged, no real safety net existed to support him or any other member of the services dealing with those issues. But ironically and unforgivably, decades later, with a support network finally in place which could and was designed to help him, Steve was denied help by the inflexible bureaucratic filter system. He slipped through the net again.

It would be seventeen years after that chance encounter in The Wellington before I became aware of the problems Steve was dealing with. As I look back now, I recognise the signs were always there.

Standing on the top of a windswept, rain-soaked mountain on a trip I never expected to take place with a friend I should never have met again, I realised that our rugby match pub conversation had set in motion a remarkable sequence of events, ultimately culminating in the creation of the Cockleshell Endeavour.

That coincidental meeting, as likely as a lottery win and in many ways as valuable, would become the catalyst for a whole series of incredible and increasingly important projects and adventures. It would steer my life and Steve's in very different directions than they were heading. It would also cement firmly in place my increasing certainty that there is no such thing as coincidence.

CHAPTER 7

BACK IN TRAINING

When we returned to the UK from our trip to the Falklands, Steve
Grenham gleefully informed me that, apart from walking the dogs,
he hadn't done any physical training in twenty-five years.

I thought he was joking. He wasn't.

Neither of us could paddle, so the immediate goal was to get
onto the water as soon as possible, start getting Steve fit again and
for us both to learn as much technique as we could as quickly as
we could.

I booked the pair of us into an outdoors centre in Anglesey for
a week's intensive training. It was the only one I could find that
was open for business in December and would accept two optimistic, middle-aged, novice kayakers for winter training on some
of the most challenging UK waterways and coastline. A brilliant
instructor called Huw Jones took us under his wing, and, without
dismissing our ambitious plans out of hand, he put us through a
tough introduction to kayaking to see what we were made of.
After some basic safety training in the pool, we moved to a freezing lake to practise our drills and embryonic kayaking techniques.
From there we set off on an expedition on the Menai Straits and
a trip through the infamous Swellies, the turbulent stretch of
water between the Britannia Bridge and the Menai Suspension
Bridge. To round off the week we took to the open sea for our first
taste of sea kayaking, it was blowing a gale, but, as Huw pointed
out, nothing to what we would likely face in the southern hemisphere. Battered, exhausted, cold and wet, and frequently under
water throughout the week, we both loved it.

Huw was pleased and not a little surprised with our progress. 'I've never taught students like you two,' he said. We took that as a complement and didn't ask him to elaborate. He also agreed to put together a training schedule to help us reach the standard we'd need to be at in the relatively short time we had. After that I created a programme to encompass Huw's training plan, as best I could with practically no budget, which would hopefully culminate in our successful circumnavigation of the Falkland Islands.

Despite the success of our initial training, the enormity of our goal soon became apparent. I contacted an American paddler who held the record for a solo circumnavigation of the islands for advice. His response: 'I had to reread your email to confirm that you actually intend to circumnavigate the Falklands in the next year, but you're both novice kayakers. I thought I'd misread it.'

He then went on, albeit very politely, to outline the scale of the challenge even to someone such as himself, a lifelong and expert paddler, and how dangerous his solo circumnavigation had proved to be. I welcomed his advice and respected what he said. The advice from everyone I approached was invaluable, if generally less than optimistic as to our chances of success. In fairness, no one dismissed us out of hand. Possibly our joint Royal Marine background along with my rowing exploits gave us at least some small level of credibility. In my defence, I hadn't been totally oblivious to the demands of such an undertaking, even at the beginning. I had enough knowledge of the sea and in particular the challenges the Southern Ocean would bring to be aware of what we were taking on. I simply had no doubt that with the right training Steve and I were more than capable of successfully overcoming the challenges. We just needed the right training.

Fitness and technique can be improved and taught. But the qualities Steve had as a young marine were still part of him. I knew he still possessed his innate strength of character – we just needed to reawaken it. The other stuff? We could put that in place along the way.

During the whole of this initial period of the Cockleshell Endeavour there was one constant along with Steve and me: Paul Rigby. Riggs, as he's known, is a former soldier in the British Army's Royal Anglian Regiment, and he's an old friend of mine. I'd got to know him many years previously through one of my best friends in the Royal Marines, Ray Amiss. Riggs had gone to school with Ray and they'd remained close friends. When I first left the marines, I lived in the same part of the country as the pair of them and we all played rugby for the same village team in Ampthill.

We remained good mates, even after my sailing work eventually took me away from the UK. When I came up with the idea of the Cockleshell Endeavour, Riggs was one of the first people I contacted for help, as I knew he was an enthusiastic paddler. From the very beginning it was a three-man effort. Without Riggs's support and constant hard work and enthusiasm, we would have achieved nothing.

In the early days of Cockleshell, Riggs would drive down to the south coast from Bedfordshire most weekends, bringing equipment and kit for us to use. He brought different kayaks for us to trial and train in on the nearby River Ouse. He helped us build the momentum at the start of the project that kept us on track to achieve our goals.

I remember pulling up with Riggs in his pickup outside Steve's house at 6 a.m. one freezing and dark Saturday December morning to pick him up for our first training run. It was an early start to make the most of the tidal flow on the Ouse. Steve answered the door bleary eyed and obviously ill prepared for the day and the conditions ahead.

It had been a long time since Steve had had to prepare for anything like what we were embarking on. It hadn't occurred to him he'd require provisions for the day or any additional clothing. That sort of planning hadn't been part of his life for a long time. To some extent Riggs and I had anticipated this, and had prepared enough rations and hot drinks for the three of us and sorted spare kit in case he was short. It still came as a shock to me and a sharp reminder that Steve would need support, certainly in the early stages as he got back into the swing of things.

With the best will in the world, it became increasingly clear it was going to take time for us to achieve the required standard as paddlers to safely attempt the circumnavigation. This was not going to be a three-month project. To keep Steve motivated and both of us on track, we needed a short-term goal to aim for.

'Fancy cracking the Devizes to Westminster, Steve?'

The Devizes to Westminster International Canoe Race takes place every Easter weekend in the UK. It's globally famous. Starting in the sleepy Wiltshire town of Devizes on the narrow confines of the Kennet and Avon Canal, the finish line is 125 miles away on the powerful tidal waters of the River Thames at Westminster Bridge, directly opposite the Houses of Parliament.

Along the route, just to make it interesting, there are seventy-one locks to negotiate, where paddlers are required to get out of their kayaks, throw the boat onto their shoulders and then run around to the other side of the lock before jumping back in the boat and paddling off. It's not for the fainthearted. It seemed the perfect fit for us.

'I'll give it a go,' Steve replied. 'What boat are we going to do it in?'

A friend, fellow ocean rower and former commando engineer Charlie Martell, had kindly loaned us his kayak, the *Black Pearl*.

She was a black canvas-skinned, collapsible folding kayak with a sturdy wooden frame; a two-man boat, bulky and slow, but stable. It was the sort of boat the Cockleshell Heroes would have used in World War II. She was forgiving of our embryonic kayaking abilities and provided the perfect platform for us to steadily adapt our bodies to the rigours of long-distance paddling.

If she had one drawback, though, it was her weight. She was a heavy piece of equipment, particularly when we had to take her out of the water and portage around any locks or obstacles. The weight issue eventually led us, rather unkindly, to give her the nickname the *Black Pig*. We would race in the *Black Pig*. Steve was thrilled . . .

With the first real goal in sight, our training steadily increased. Most weekends during the winter we were on the River Ouse, whatever the weather. Our lack of technique compensated for by the sturdy and seemingly unsinkable *Black Pig*, week after week we ground out increasingly greater and occasionally swifter mileage. The conditions were often wet, frequently windy and always cold. On more than one occasion, all of the above.

Even early on it was obvious the effect the routine and challenge was having on Steve. He was loving it. Obviously blessed with good genes, Steve's twenty-five-year sabbatical from any kind of meaningful physical activity seemed to have had little lingering impact on his capabilities. Whatever he lacked in technique in a kayak, he more than made up for in straight-line speed. He was a powerful paddler and a natural long-distance racer. More importantly, it was obvious he was enjoying and thriving on the challenge. As much as we were setting ourselves goals to achieve like the Devizes to Westminster and ultimately a circumnavigation of the Falkland Islands, our only real aim was to help Steve back on the road to recovery. It became clear quite early on that Steve was on that road.

CHAPTER 8

CHARITY STARTS AT HOME

When the Cockleshell Endeavour project was created, one of our main aims beyond Steve Grenham's recovery was to raise awareness of the issues of PTSD, the condition he was struggling with. It was logical that to help achieve that aim we should link with a military charity.

When I left the Royal Marines, I worked for almost five years as a personal chauffeur for Paul Orchard-Lisle, the senior partner of an international real estate company in London. It was a great job and I only left to pursue my long-held sailing ambitions. Despite my many shortcomings as a chauffeur, I remained in touch with my old boss and occasionally we'd meet up for lunch, as we still do. Maybe my replacement writing off his Aston Martin and a large chunk of a local pub 'avoiding a fox' a few months after my departure painted me in a much better light than I may have deserved.

Paul was the first person I turned to for advice about attracting support from the corporate market when I decided to row the Atlantic in 2001. That project and every one since has benefited from Paul Orchard-Lisle's support to some degree. Inadvertently, I think I may have become his most expensive chauffeur, despite the best efforts of my fox-avoiding successor.

When the Cockleshell Endeavour began over a decade later, once more he was the first person I approached for advice. He informed me that I was obviously still bonkers, but it was encouraging that I seemed to have at least moved on from ocean rowing boats at long last.

Paul introduced me to Keith Breslauer, managing director of Patron Capital, a financial investment company that he'd built. Although an American, Keith has formed a remarkably close bond with the Royal Marines. His company directly contributes to the Royal Marine Charity, but his involvement goes far beyond that. He organises and sponsors the largest annual fundraising event each year for the corps, The Royal Marines Commando Dinner held at the Guildhall in London. It's an event that raises close to, and in 2018 in excess of, one million pounds for the charity every year. Patron provide job placements for recovering veterans, and Keith has become a force of nature in championing the Royal Marines and their charity.

We seemed to hit it off at our first meeting, which was scheduled for twenty minutes but went on for twice that. Keith appeared genuinely fascinated with my ocean rowing adventures, particularly the story of my sinking in the North Pacific, surviving by the skin of my teeth and then choosing to go back and try again. As well as being an incredibly successful businessman, Keith is also a highly accomplished mountaineer and skier – I think because of that he recognised at least something in my passion for the ocean.

When I got around to talking about the Cockleshell Endeavour project and what I was aiming to achieve, he was even more interested.

'How are you not connected with the Royal Marines on any of this?' he finally asked.

I'd contacted the corps in 2000, during the preparation for the first Atlantic row with my brother Steve, also a former Royal Marine. As luck would have it, bad in this case, two serving Royal Marines, Tim Welford and Dom Mee, guys who would one day become great friends of mine, were preparing to row the North Pacific at that precise time. All the Royal Navy's efforts let alone the corps were being directed at supporting them and promoting their project. There was no interest or capacity in supporting two former marines, brothers or otherwise, in an Atlantic rowing project. It was a case of unfortunate timing, but I never approached the corps for support again. I explained all this to Keith.

'Patron are going to support your project for sure. We'll provide some sponsorship for the Cockleshell Endeavour. However, I'm going to do more than that. I'm going to reconnect you with the corps. There's such a resource of guys like you out there doing incredible stuff like this, but the corps aren't picking up on that. They can help you and you are a great advert for them. I'm going to reintroduce you to your family again, Mick,' he said, laughing.

Keith had picked up on something I've touched on before: there is a vast number of former marines, and almost all regard themselves still very much a part of the Royal Marine family. There was simply a disconnect from the serving marines and those who'd left. Everyone knew that bond existed, but everyone was guilty of taking it for granted. More importantly, everyone was guilty of failing to see its value. With the possible exception of Keith Breslauer.

It was ironic that it took an American civilian to recognise that fact. He saw before anyone else the intrinsic value the wider Royal Marine family brought to the serving corps.

'You need to get connected with The Royal Marines Charity too,' he said, as we shook hands at the end of our meeting.

A week later, true to his word, Keith arranged a meeting for me with Jonathan Ball, a former Royal Marine officer and now one of the senior figures in the charity. Jonathan immediately provided me with several contacts who could potentially be of help to Steve with his recovery. He was also keen to explore ways for the charity to connect with the project and develop ways to promote both the work the charity was doing and what we were trying to achieve with the Cockleshell Endeavour. It was a breath of fresh air, and felt like the start of a partnership.

It was. It was the start of a connection which continues to this day through all of the Cockleshell Endeavour projects. The Royal Marines Charity has supported every project we've undertaken. It's an honour to have that connection with them and to be able to raise money for the continued invaluable work they do. It was one of many things I would have to thank Keith Breslauer for over the coming years.

CHAPTER 9

DEVIZES TO WESTMINSTER

The three months leading up to the Devizes race had gone well. With Riggs's invaluable help, training had been consistent and largely successful. Most importantly, Steve was enjoying the process. To such an extent that he didn't feel the need to go back to the charity he'd approached about his PTSD for the formal diagnosis. I felt he may have still resented the door being closed in his face at the first approach; whatever the reasoning behind it, it was his decision to make. Although we were still by no means great technical paddlers, we were much fitter and stronger. In truth the technical demands of paddling a folding kayak in the Devizes to Westminster are not that great. It really comes down to a stubborn determination to keep going. Fortunately for us, at that point, stubborn determination was one of the few strengths we possessed.

Riggs, who'd not only supported all our training efforts but also trained alongside us in his own sea kayak, had decided to enter the race himself as a solo kayaker. His plan was to finish the course totally unsupported, taking everything he would require for the three days on board and with no team to help him. It meant his already bulky sea kayak was even heavier, laden down with camping gear and all the supplies and kit he would require. He would be much slower than the other super light solo racing boats taking part.

It also meant at each of the seventy-one locks he would be dragging a boat which weighed almost as much as the other boats with the paddler still inside them. In layman's terms, he was taking part in a Formula 1 race in a camper van. It seemed, much like me and Steve, Riggs liked a challenge.

In the run up to the Devizes the three of us took part in a few of the warm-up races which covered different sections of the full course. These were designed to increase our familiarity with the route and work out our likely pace, so as to accurately predict our arrival time at Teddington's tidal lock.

The beginning of one of these practice races was on a stretch of the waterway wide enough for a mass start. Competitors jockeyed for position along a notional line across the river, excitement building, everyone desperate to be as close to the start line as possible when the official signalled, but careful not to cross it too early.

Well aware we could become an unwanted obstacle for the other, swifter race competitors, Steve and I and Riggs held back from that frantic melee. We calmly paddled across the line a minute or two after the swarm of other competitors had sped off.

In this race we were very much the tortoises to their hares, and our agendas very different. For us it was all about completion, not how fast. Thirty-two miles later, Steve and I crossed the finish line. Riggs would come in just under an hour after us and all of us several hours after the bulk of the other racers in their super-light state-of-the-art racing boats, many of whom were already packed up and on their way home by the time we finished. Despite that inevitable result, it had been a great training run for us all and an invaluable day's experience on the race route. Although tired, we were happy. We would be even happier twenty-four hours later.

I checked online the next day to confirm our times on the race website. I opened the results section at the top of the solo kayaker's page and the name Paul Rigby was at the top of the list. Next to it was the phrase: First in Class. I scrolled down in disbelief, thinking it was a mistake, but in fact every one of the super-fast paddlers who'd left both our boats for dead at the start were placed behind him. Then I noticed an asterisk and an explanation. All of those hair-triggered solo boats had crossed the start line before the starter's signal and they'd all been disqualified. Riggs had been the only solo kayaker to cross the start line after the signal. We took it as a good omen.

Come Easter bank holiday weekend, April 2015, it was time for the Devizes to Westminster itself. Riggs had set off a day earlier with the rest of the solo competitors racing over three days. We started on the Saturday morning, and if all went well we'd reach the finish line at Westminster Bridge sometime on Sunday afternoon.

The night before the race we travelled up to Devizes so we'd be ready for an early morning start. We'd worked out the best time for us to leave to reach the last lock before the tidal stretch of the Thames at Teddington. This was key, because if you arrived at the wrong state of the tide you could be stranded at Teddington for a very long time. It could put hours on your finish time and possibly lead to you not finishing at all.

As dawn broke the following morning, we arrived at the start line. Everything progressed relatively smoothly completing the safety briefs and kit inspections. We carefully lowered the *Black Pig*, our home for the next two days, onto the tight confines of the narrow canal and gingerly stepped into the two paddling positions, me forwards and Steve directly behind. Then, after a few minutes final preparation, we pushed off, taking the first tentative strokes of our first genuine kayaking challenge. If the Cockleshell Endeavour had been born on the summit of Mount Harriet, this was its first day at school.

The canal is so narrow at the start that each team sets off single file. With the cheers of our support team ringing out from the bank, Steve and I took our first competitive strokes in the *Black Pig* beneath the picturesque bridge and began our race to London. Next stop Westminster Bridge and the Houses of Parliament, 125 miles away.

To succeed in the Devizes to Westminster race most competitors need a support team providing food and drink along the whole length of the route, not to mention a healthy dose of encouragement. We had a phenomenal support team.

Steve's brother Tony was the first to offer his services, along with Phil Booth, whose house we'd stayed at the night prior to the race start. Phil had known the Grenhams most of his life and was more than just a friend of the family. Considered another brother by Tony and Steve, another son by Mrs G., he'd lived with them for several years after his family chose to emigrate when he was about to take his exams. Like Riggs, he'd decided to enlist in the army when he left school, although unlike Riggs, who chose the infantry, Phil joined the Royal Tank Regiment. He drove a Challenger battle tank in the first Gulf War, fighting in Kuwait and Iraq.

Ric Strange, an old friend of mine from the Royal Marines, also came on board, helping in the first training races on the course and then the race itself. I've been great friends with Ric since the early 1980s, sharing a house with him for a couple of years at one point and serving for even more years together in the same troop. A former marine of a much more recent vintage, Si Reed, also volunteered his services. Si's an accomplished paddler who'd started to help out with some of our preparation immediately before the race. I'd met him a few years earlier, when we were both working together as armed security on anti-piracy escorts in the

Red Sea and Indian Ocean, protecting commercial shipping from Somali pirates.

Everybody but Steve's brother Tony was ex-armed forces. Without having to ask anyone directly, a support team had formed naturally around the project. I didn't realise it at the time, but this was the first example of the lifeblood which would eventually run through every challenge we undertook with the Cockleshell Endeavour. People wanted to help.

The simple reason was the family ethos that binds service personnel together, regardless of their background. The armed forces are the one place in modern society where the values which close-knit families exhibit are demonstrated and, more importantly, expected.

Ric and Si's help, Riggs's support and perhaps even my own actions were because we reacted to the situation like family. Riggs's initial and instinctive response when I approached him in the beginning was: 'How can I help?' It became the byword for everything we did. From the confines of the Kennet and Avon Canal at the start to the rugged coastline of the Falkland Islands and on to the vast expanse of the Pacific Ocean, that ethos of family, of 'How can I help?', would become the central theme which ran through all of the Cockleshell Endeavour projects.

Our support family formed themselves into two teams and planned a schedule that allowed them to leapfrog one another along the route, so at least one team would always be in place with food and drink at any designated point as we approached.

Ric told me he'd decided to cycle the course next to us, along the canal towpath, which he confidently informed me 'runs pretty much the length of the whole route'.

There was a flaw in his plan, though. Several days of rain leading up to the event reduced the canal tow path to a boggy track, and the hybrid bike he chose was definitely not the ideal one for the job. Only a few miles into the race, making our way steadily along the narrow canal, and our 'peddling' partner had apparently disappeared. The next time we saw him was at the feed stop several miles further along the canal. By then he'd given up on his bike, which had ground to a halt in the glutinous mud, and he'd hopped, crestfallen, into one of our two leapfrogging mobile support vans to help out during the rest of the race.

As the first day slipped into the evening, our bodies were steadily, if at times reluctantly, getting used to the increasing workload. We were now in uncharted territory in both miles through the water and hours on it. None of our training runs had taken us beyond thirty-four miles. We were also slowly chalking off the exhausting portages around the many locks that give the race it's unique identity.

As uncharted as the territory was in terms of kayaking, it was not uncharted in terms of endurance. Royal Marine training and operations are built on physical and mental endurance. You don't have to be Superman, but you do have to be able to keep going. As the night closed in around us and the canal banks, trees and hedges merged into the dark, it was apparent that both of us still retained a certain level of endurance to go with the innate stubborn determination we were relying on to get to the finish. We were having no problems keeping going.

There was little we couldn't find humour in, despite the workload, constant discomfort and growing fatigue. Most importantly, we were working well as a team. We were maintaining a steady pace through the portages and our speed through the water seemed reasonable. Things were going well.

At about 2 a.m. we pulled over to the bank for a food stop in the pitch black. Tony came over and handed us both some snacks to keep us going. 'You're doing really well, guys, you're second in class. There's only one team in front of you and apparently they're the SAS team. You've already passed a para team and two boats in your class have already dropped out.'

We were almost speechless. As we paddled back out into the darkness, for the first time we began to consider we might be capable of more than just finishing the race. We were doing fine mentally and physically, and paddling and negotiating the challenging portages were well within our capabilities. Could we up the pace and catch the team in front?

The conditions for the race that year were good. Despite the heavy rain, which had fallen in the days preceding the start, only brief showers affected us during the race itself. There was unfortunately, though, no great flow of water on the canal towards the lock at Teddington to help us on our way. The wind, what little of it there was, also brought little advantage as it steadfastly refused to fill in behind and help us. Every mile of progress was earned solely with the paddles. It was a long and hard night's work in our trusty *Black Pig*, punctuated with episodes of hallucination and confusion as the darkness combined with fatigue and lack of sleep to scramble our senses.

'How long did you do this shit for on your rowing boat again, Mick?' Steve asked me at one point during the night.

'One hundred and eighty-nine days, ten hours and fifty-five minutes.'

'Fuck me, you must be mad. One night and I'm going nuts!'

'You could make tea on my rowing boat,' I said. 'And there was somewhere to sleep.'

'Yeah, that would make all the difference,' he quipped, continuing to paddle.

I was glad that we were still managing to see the funny side of things as the race began to take its toll. One of my main concerns throughout the whole project was that my friendship with Steve should not be wrecked by what we were doing. There are a number of factors to consider with PTSD and mental health issues, none of which I was aware of at the beginning of our adventures.

Once, before I knew of Steve's battles with the effects of PTSD, we'd been walking to a pub on a night out. A car had been pulled over by the police at the side of the road. Two police officers were in the process of breathalysing the driver. I'm not sure which if any offence had been committed but the driver didn't seem overly concerned and it appeared routine and nothing to get excited about.

Except Steve did get excited.

Completely out of character and from nowhere, his mood swung and he began remonstrating with one of the police officers. There was no reason for Steve's reaction. It was nothing to do with us. It made no sense and I'd never seen him react to such an innocuous situation so aggressively before. He was telling the police officers to 'leave people alone!' and stop 'fucking people's lives up'. It didn't make any sense. Steve is an imposing figure and the two police officers thankfully reacted very calmly and professionally. It could easily have escalated out of control if they hadn't. One officer dealt with the car driver while the other calmly spoke to Steve, asking him to carry on on his way. That didn't seem to help, though. If anything, it made him worse.

I stepped in before it got out of hand. 'We're too old for this kind of nonsense, mate. Let's go. They're just doing their job, it's got nothing to do with us.' The advice seemed to have a little more effect coming from me. The confrontation evaporated as quickly as it had begun, and a second later Steve and I were walking towards the next pub like nothing had happened.

I had no idea then, as it just seemed like an isolated overreaction after a couple of beers, but massive mood swings and resentment towards authority can be an indicator of mental health issues.

The next time I saw an example of that kind of reaction from Steve, I was a little more aware. It's as well I was, as I'd be on the end of it.

Riggs and I had arrived at Steve's house to pick him up for training early one Saturday morning. It was January, a month into training, freezing cold and dark. I'd been busy trying to raise sponsorship and support for the project, with limited success. Happily, I had good news. The Brighton branch of Fitness First had agreed to provide us with free membership for the duration of the Cockleshell Endeavour. It was a very positive step in terms of training and would also be a big help with the budget and PR. I was pleased.

Steve was tired when he came to the door and I immediately handed him the forms we both needed to sign. In hindsight I should have mentioned it later. It wasn't the right time. I wasn't thinking, just pleased to have positive news.

'What's this?' he asked, curious and a little irritated.

'Forms for membership of Fitness First, mate. They've agreed to sponsor us.'

'Fuck that,' he replied instantly. 'I'm not poncing around on a treadmill with a bunch of poseurs. I'm not going.'

Sponsorship was proving tough to come by, so having one of the first successes so roundly thrown back in my face pissed me off. 'I don't give a fuck if you go there, just fill the form in so we can accept the sponsorship.'

I thrust the forms towards him in the doorway. He promptly grabbed them and threw them back at me.

'Fuck your forms and fuck your kayaking! I don't need you or anybody else telling me what to do.' He slammed the door violently, leaving me picking up the sponsorship forms on the doorstep.

I walked back to Riggs, who was sitting in his truck blissfully unaware of what had happened.

'Is Steve ready?' he asked.

'Not exactly, mate.'

I gave it a few minutes, hoping he'd calm down and come and join us. He didn't. I went back and knocked on the door. Steve eventually answered.

'I thought you two had gone,' he said.

'Not a lot of point us kayaking without you, is there?' I answered. 'Get your kit. No point ruining the day because of a stupid argument. It would be a waste of sandwiches, mate.'

He grabbed his paddling kit and we joined Riggs in the truck. That was the end of the matter – the anger gone as quickly as it arrived.

That incident had served as a timely reminder for me that we weren't just creating a kayaking project with the Cockleshell Endeavour. The kayaking was the tool we were using to deal with the real goal, helping Steve on the road to recovery. The kayaking was incidental, just a means to an end. Its positive effect on Steve was all that mattered. I needed to bear that in mind, and I needed to bear in mind how I approached situations in the future.

The last thing Steve wanted at that point was anyone telling him what to do, least of all his mate. Sudden mood swings and anger towards any form of perceived authority were his natural defences. If I didn't want to lose a mate and, in the process, lose the chance to help him, I'd have to learn quickly how to manage those problems more effectively. I'm glad to say that the one constant theme throughout all of our paddling exploits was the steady improvement in Steve, mentally and physically. The mood swings and loss of temper, which even at the beginning were isolated and out of character, diminished and ultimately disappeared. His self-confidence and belief grew in direct proportion to his increasing fitness and our progress on the water.

Back on the river, as the long black night was thankfully finally swallowed by the dawn, we approached a stretch of the course we weren't familiar with. We also approached our first real problem in the race: we seemed to have lost our support team. With the sun and temperature steadily rising, the previous two stops where we could have expected a resupply of provisions had been worryingly empty. No support team and no resupply. We were nearly out of water and we were totally out of food. Our energy levels were starting to flag.

'What's happened to The A-Team?' Steve asked, The A-Team being the title we'd given them, hearkening to the TV show of our youth.

'No idea, mate. I'm sure they'll be up ahead somewhere soon.'

They weren't. It was several hours and a couple more missed stops in the increasing heat before we saw them again.

'Where have you been?' Steve shouted out as we approached the bank.

'We missed you by minutes at the last couple of stops,' Tony shouted back. 'You'd just gone through as we arrived.'

'Likely story, you've been getting your fat heads down in the car,' Steve replied.

'No we haven't. You went the wrong way – you've done an extra three or four miles. We've been trying to work out where you were.'

'The wrong way?' I said.

'Yep. There're two options at a place called Ham Island. You two took the wrong option.'

In the early hours, exhausted and struggling with the lack of sleep on a stretch of the river we weren't familiar with, we'd apparently paddled past a fork in the river and added a few extra miles to the course.

'Bollocks!' we both said in annoyed frustration.

Any chance of an unlikely victory in the folding kayak class of the race had all but disappeared. We still managed to close the two-hour gap on the eventual winners, despite the additional miles we'd inadvertently paddled. But catching up and pipping them at the post was too much to ask.

We were still on track to complete our original goal, though. We were going to successfully finish the Devizes to Westminster kayak race. What's more, we were going to finish it in a boat that was almost certainly the heaviest taking part.

Paddling, exhausted, aching and desperate for sleep, we made our way along the final miles of the Thames and through the increasingly familiar architecture of London. The fast-flowing tidal water was driving us towards our goal. We were both desperate to reach the finish line and step ashore at Westminster Bridge. Even the bulky *Black Pig* now seemed fragile and vulnerable on the comparatively vast waters of the River Thames. It seemed a long time since the cramped confines at the start line on the Kennet and Avon Canal at Devizes.

Frustratingly, the last and swiftest miles of the race seemed to drag the most. Westminster Bridge seemed to take for ever to come into view. When it did, though, it was an amazing and welcome sight. As well as the hundreds of tourists milling around, there were dozens of race supporters, and there on the bridge overlooking the steps which served as our finish line was the Grenham family. We spotted Steve's wonderful wife, Aicha, his brother Tony and Tony's partner Jodi, Phil Booth and of course the guys from the A-Team who'd helped us get there. Most noticeable of all, though, was Steve's mum, Mrs G., beaming from ear to ear and waving and cheering.

We paddled up to the stairway that led down to the water's edge from the south bank of the river and onto a small quay awash at the base of it. Two guys standing in the murky waters of the Thames in drysuits caught our boat and grabbed hold of us to keep us steady. They then expertly helped us out and onto the quay. Steve and I turned to take the *Black Pig* from them.

'No, no,' one of the guys said, 'don't worry, we'll get it up to the top for you. You boys are finished.'

He turned back to pick up our trusty kayak with his colleague and all I heard as I mounted the stairway was, 'Bloody hell! This weighs a tonne! Can we have a hand here?'

I smiled knowingly and followed Steve up the steps slowly. More stewards and volunteers from the race helped us ascend safely. At the top we were stopped with a handshake and a medal on a ribbon was placed around our necks. We'd done it! We'd completed the Devizes to Westminster International Canoe Race. Not only that, but somehow we'd managed to finish second in class.

Steve's family engulfed him, everyone delighted, patting him on the back. Steve was equally as happy. It was a privilege to be part of such a great family moment. As the excitement died down and Steve headed off to have a shower and put some dry clothes on, Mrs G. and Tony were standing in front of me chatting. Mrs G., almost in tears, turned and said to nobody in particular, 'I'm so proud, so proud. I've never been prouder of him not since he came back from the Falklands.'

I'd be lying if I didn't admit to feeling a lump in my throat when I heard those words. Mrs G. was the catalyst for the whole Cockleshell Endeavour project. It was her concern for Steve that had been behind our return to the Falklands. She'd been worried for a long time that she was losing her son to a toxic, creeping mental illness. At the end of the Devizes to Westminster race I think she realised he'd turned a corner.

For me, there's nothing we've achieved since with the Cockleshell Endeavour which eclipses that moment at Westminster Bridge. Mrs G.'s reaction and the Grenham family welcome was a very special moment. There could be no greater endorsement of what we were trying to achieve. Sadly, it has even greater significance now as, tragically, Mrs G. passed away in June 2016. She would never see Steve deliver on his promise to circumnavigate the Falkland Islands. I like to think that sadness and loss is tempered by the fact Mrs G. and Steve knew she'd already got her son back.

CHAPTER 10

HIGHLAND STORMS

After the success of the Devizes to Westminster race, Steve Grenham and I looked for the next challenge to keep us on track for our return to the Falkland Islands.

'How about going up to Scotland and cracking the Caledonian Canal?' Riggs suggested. 'I did it with a mate a couple of years ago. It was great.'

The Caledonian Canal stretches from Fort William to Inverness, connecting the west and east coasts of Scotland. Sixty miles long, it's a combination of man-made waterways and four Scottish lochs, including Loch Ness, complete with mythical monster. It links the opposing coastlines of Scotland through the spectacularly beautiful Scottish Highlands along what's known as the Great Glen.

Originally planned for the use of small commercial vessels and fishing boats when the canal was opened in 1822, in modern times it achieved the status of a scheduled ancient monument and attracts more than half a million visitors a year. Some of them are kayakers.

Fort William had significance for us: it was close to Achnacarry, which was the training centre for commandos during World War II. The commandos had been formed on Churchill's orders in 1940, specifically to take the war back to the then all-conquering German army in Europe. He wanted to regain the initiative by carrying out a series of innovative, courageous and morale boosting raids on the occupied and heavily fortified European coastline – 1700 commandos would eventually pay the ultimate price for those actions, with many more seriously wounded. However, the value of those raids from a morale-boosting perspective was immeasurable. They gave the British public their first victories against the seemingly unstoppable German war machine. They signalled a crucial turning point in the momentum of World War II and gave people hope. The Royal Marines now proudly fulfils the United Kingdom's commando role; so, what better place for two former Royal Marines to start and finish our next adventure.

Si Reed, one of the A-Team who supported our Devizes to Westminster effort, offered to join Steve, me and Riggs. The plan was to complete the paddle over four days, camping overnight at various stops along the route. It'd be two days to Inverness then two days heading back.

It was May 2015 and the paddle out from Fort William was spectacular. The weather was fine, the paddling relaxed and enjoyable, particularly after the physical and mental challenges of the Devizes. We were using solo kayaks hired locally, which made logistics for the trip much simpler. The Scottish countryside was breathtakingly beautiful; the Great Glen cutting a narrow path through the dramatic highland landscape. Clear blue skies contrasted against the vivid green of the steep and imposing hills and mountains that bordered much of our route, particularly the sections through the lochs. In places, on the narrower connecting canal sections, dense woodland encroached to the water's edge and there wasn't a breath of wind, with just the sound of our paddle strokes and deer calling to break the silence. We could not have asked for two better days as we arrived at the halfway point of our journey, Inverness. We posed for pictures on the final lock, which was all that separated the canal from the North Sea on the Scottish east coast. Then we turned our kayaks around and began heading back the way we'd come.

Conditions now became very different. A low-pressure area had formed, bringing with it cooler weather, ominously grey skies, rain and strong headwinds.

As we reached Loch Ness it was clear the twenty-three miles that stretched before us were going to be a lot more challenging than the original journey east. Loch Ness is deceptively large, despite being an inland waterway, and in bad weather conditions it can be a very dangerous stretch of water, particularly in a kayak. It's apparently the only stretch of inland waterway with a dedicated Royal National Lifeboat Institute station.

The water, cold year round, now seemed freezing, with the strong winds blowing directly into our faces. The waves the wind created soaked us as we fought our way through them. The summer-like weather of the previous two days was now long gone. We battled our way along the northern edge of the loch, hoping to gain at least some respite from the wind and waves by staying as close as we could to the shore.

Steve, a naturally fast straight-line paddler, had a different model of boat from the rest of us and it soon became clear he was even quicker than normal in it. For the first time it also became apparent Steve was either unable or unwilling to work as a team when we were in solo kayaks. It was a worrying discovery. He'd see the target ahead of him, get his head down and power towards it, everything and everyone else forgotten. His determination and courage were commendable qualities, but the possible consequences if things went wrong were a worry for me.

With the exception of Si Reed, who was an accomplished paddler, none of us were proficient enough to reliably deal with emergencies on our own at that stage. Even on the lochs it was crucial that all four of us stayed close to cope with any possible emergency in the worsening conditions. In the Falklands, where there would just be me and Steve at the mercy of the islands'

61

notoriously unpredictable weather and the ferocious Southern Ocean, it could prove fatal to both of us if we became separated.

As we approached a northerly bulge in the predominantly long and thin Loch Ness, a few miles before Urquhart Castle, the wind veered viciously. The temperature and topography created a localised katabatic wind which swept down from the mountains, twisting the prevailing wind direction from head on to beam (side) on. Steve was already some way in front of the three of us, and as this wind hit he simply powered directly across the widening stretch of water ahead of us into ominously building breaking waves. There was a real risk of capsize. We shouted out to Steve to stop, but he was oblivious to our calls. He was head down and making for the silhouette of the castle which had come into view on the distant headland.

We should have and would have stopped to wait out the sudden change of conditions had we been able to prevent Steve from forging ahead. Now that he'd committed to the crossing there was no way we could leave him. The three of us contoured slightly north around the bulge, trying to limit our exposure to the building waves by hugging the shore as much as we could. In doing so it meant we took a slightly longer route. Worryingly, because of the worsening weather and the distance he was putting between us, we lost sight of Steve.

It's barely two miles across that stretch of water on Loch Ness. It felt like the longest two miles I'd ever paddled. From the moment we lost sight of Steve I was conscious that, if he capsized, he would be in serious trouble. He'd be blown away from us by the driving wind and we'd have little chance of locating him. Hypothermia could prove fatal in minutes in the freezing water of the loch. We'd learned and practised techniques to get back in the boat alone after a capsize, but in the bitter cold conditions, with formidable waves, it would be an incredibly difficult manoeuvre.

I was angry he'd ploughed on into trouble without any consideration and without us, but at the same time I was worried sick.

By the time the three of us paddled up to the shoreline beneath the castle, less than an hour later, the wind had dropped, the sun had returned and it felt like a different day. Having beached his kayak, Steve was lying on the shoreline eating a protein bar, oblivious to our concerns.

'Why didn't you wait when we shouted?' I asked, any anger being replaced by relief, but I was also conscious of not provoking an argument.

'I didn't hear any shouting,' he replied.

'What if you'd gone over?' I asked.

'If I'd stopped, I would have capsized. I had no choice. I just needed to get to the other side,' he said, seemingly unaware of the potential for disaster he'd just skirted.

'What if one of us had capsized?' I asked.

'There were three of you, you'd have been fine.' He seemed unconcerned.

Steve's blunt and dismissive reaction was partly down to his lack of awareness. He didn't appreciate many of the dangers that threatened on open water in deteriorating conditions. Some of that reaction, however, was down to the issues he was coping with every day relating to PTSD. I'd become aware over the months working with him that he treated any serious problem or challenge as a threat – he faced it head on and smashed through it, whatever it was. There was little scope for reasoning. He just dealt with what was in front of him as fast as he could.

Consequences didn't come into the equation. He covered any lack of confidence or fear with aggression and courage. He had no real concern for himself at that point, so why should I expect him to have any concern for me or for anyone else. One of the most gratifying things which would eventually emerge from the whole Cockleshell Endeavour experience was to witness how steadily that mentality in Steve completely reversed.

To cope with Steve's reluctance or inability to function reliably in a team, I needed to be a far superior kayaker than I was. I needed to be able to approach the project as if I were paddling alone, but also so I could become Steve's support team, independent of him. I was nowhere near that level of kayaking skill.

Once more I had to remind myself that the aim of what we were trying to achieve wasn't based on the kayaking goals; it was to get Steve back on track physically and mentally. I needed to find a way forwards where we could achieve that goal despite any shortcoming we may have as kayakers. After Scotland, doubts formed in my mind.

In an ideal world, any shortcoming we had as paddlers could be addressed with more training. We just needed time and training to reach the standard.

We needed another challenge.

CHAPTER 11

THE RACE TO THE MIDNIGHT SUN

The Yukon River Quest in Canada is the longest annual kayak race in the world. It is 444 miles and three days of almost non-stop paddling, from the Yukon state capital Whitehorse to Dawson City. Steve, Si, Riggs and I planned to take part in June 2015, and it promised to be the Caledonian Canal and Devizes to Westminster rolled into one.

There were no lock gates on the Yukon to negotiate, just freezing fast-flowing water, white-water rapids, the threat of grizzly bears and three days and nights in the kayaks. Considering neither of us had paddled a stroke in a kayak until barely six months previously, our learning curve along with our optimism seemed to show no sign of tapering off.

Our training in advance of the Yukon remained consistent; as much time as possible spent on the local rivers in Sussex grinding the miles out and venturing onto the sea to improve our skills whenever the weather permitted. On race day we lined up with fifty-three other teams on the start line. There were solo and tandem kayaks and canoes taking part, along with larger open boats with crews of up to eight people on board. There was a Le Mans-style racing start down to the shoreline, where our boats were waiting for us to push off onto the Yukon and begin our journey.

My build up to the start had gone less than smoothly. Thirty minutes before the starting gun, I had been foolishly slicing a piece of tape with an open blade so I could attach a small emergency pack to my flotation device. I wasn't paying full attention, the knife slipped and I put an inch-long gash directly across the web of my left hand between the thumb and forefinger. Blood was spurting everywhere. It was the definition of a schoolboy error! I covered the wound, put some pressure on it and, cursing my stupidity, looked around for somewhere to grab a bandage from. I eventually wandered into the nearby museum where a helpful if rather horrified curator supplied me with a first aid box. Fifteen minutes later I re-emerged with an ungainly dressing in place on a throbbing left hand along with a box of painkillers. The cut couldn't have been in a less helpful place.

I'd soon discover things were going to get even worse.

Less than a mile along the Yukon in our respective kayaks, with the race in full flow, my paddle unexpectedly and alarmingly came apart. One half of the paddle wound up in each of my hands. The locking button connecting the separate sections halfway along the shaft had chosen to disintegrate. We had been one of the last teams to sign up for the race and one of the last teams to arrive in Whitehorse. The kayaks and the kit we collected from the rental shop were basically what they had left. Take it or leave it. I was now paying the price.

As boats streamed past me, I looked desperately for a quick fix. I had a spare paddle, but it was difficult to reach and not as light or as efficient as the broken one. I grabbed some snack bars I'd taped to the inside of my cockpit and peeled off the masking tape I'd used to secure them there. Pushing the paddle together again I wrapped the tape around the shaft of my paddle where the two halves locked together. It wasn't ideal but it seemed to work. The paddle remained in one piece and seemed solid enough. I wrapped an additional strip of tape around the top of the joint, just to make sure, then gingerly began to paddle again. It was working fine.

So, with my left hand still throbbing angrily, wrapped in a hastily applied bandage, and my paddle now held together with strips of tape, I headed off in pursuit of the rest of my teammates on our journey to Dawson. It certainly hadn't been the start I'd anticipated.

We settled down to the first night's kayaking in the disorientating twilight of the land of midnight sun. The teams were already stretching out over the length of the course, each one settling into their own pace. I hadn't seen Steve or Si since my problem with the paddle. I'd discover later they were paddling on ahead together, maintaining a consistent and fast pace. Steve, a strong straight-line paddler, was in his element in the race. Si, a highly proficient paddler in a sleek and competitive racing kayak, was beginning to realise he was taking part in an event he might actually be able to win or at least podium.

I'd also lost sight of Riggs at the start, and presumed he was either with Steve and Si, or somewhere ahead between them and me. I'd spent most of the day paddling as hard as I could in the vain hope of catching up with at least one of my team members, however unlikely that seemed.

Lake Labarge is the first major challenge in the race. Just a few hours out from Whitehorse, it's where the Yukon River widens into an expansive stretch of water thirty-one miles long. Notorious for its unpredictable and challenging weather, it is also devoid of any helpful flow of current. Unlike the rest of the Yukon river, every mile on Lake Labarge is earned. The key to the race can be reaching and escaping the lake as swiftly as possible. After a long day paddling, I finally said goodbye to Labarge at its northern most tip, rejoining the reassuringly fast-flowing tighter confines of the Yukon. It was an enormous relief to finally say farewell to the lake and rejoin the rapidly moving river. Just before I reached that point, though, I heard a voice behind shouting my name.

'Mick! Mick!'

I turned to look, and saw Riggs paddling up to join me with a beaming grin on his face. Apparently, he'd been behind me the whole time I'd been navigating the lake, but steadily gaining on me. It was great to see a familiar face. The remaining two days paddling, which I had been anticipating completing alone, now took on a new complexion. I'd have company, which would make all the difference.

As midnight approached, and with the eerie twilight of the Yukon summer nights engulfing us for the first time, the current picked up its pace. As we came around what amounted to a hairpin bend in the river I saw and heard a bank of white water ahead. There appeared to be a shallow ledge just beneath the surface of the water stretching out into the river, creating a large area of turbulent, rough water. There was a safe route around it, but as I headed towards that safe passage, I saw another boat heading directly into the steep standing waves. I wasn't certain but it looked like it was capsized. The unfortunate paddler was directly ahead of me, but behind Riggs.

I managed to pull up just behind the figure in the water, clinging to the upturned hull of his boat. It was a man – a very big man – and he was in trouble. He'd capsized in freezing water in the middle of the night and was apparently unable to self-right his boat. He wasn't even attempting to get the boat upright again, just clinging on for dear life. To make matters worse, at least for him, the only person in a position to rescue him appeared to be me, one of the least experienced kayakers on the water.

I paddled my boat closer to the semi-submerged hull and assessed the situation as best I could. It was a solo Canadian kayak, an open boat that you power with a single bladed paddle using alternate strokes, either side of the kayak. If it had been a classic kayak design like mine, I could easily have helped the guy self-right the boat and get him back inside it, even in the fast-moving freezing water. Steve and I had practised this technique many times and had become highly proficient at it.

I had no experience with Canadian kayaks, though, and the river was far too cold for me to start experimenting with solutions now. The clock was ticking on how long this guy could function in the bitterly cold water. I needed to get him out quickly.

'I'm going to pull up alongside you now, mate,' I said, sounding confident, while feeling decidedly less so. 'Hold on to your boat and grab hold of mine with your other hand and I'll paddle us to the shore.'

With him acting as a human bridge between my boat and his, I desperately struck out for the shore. The water was racing through that stretch of the river, funnelled by the tight turns and shallows. As soon as I got anywhere near the shore the boat touched the shallowing bottom, spun around in the ferocious current and we were dragged, spinning, back into the middle of the river. I was lucky I didn't capsize. I tried again with the same result. My friend in the water was getting colder by the minute and even more fatigued. 'I'm freezing, please get me out.'

'Don't worry, mate,' I said brightly. 'Third time lucky.'

I was becoming increasingly anxious. What if I wasn't capable of getting him safely to the shore?

Then there was an enormous stroke of luck. Ahead of us in the twilight I could see a tiny, low lying island in the middle of the river. This would surely be easier to paddle onto than the edge of the fast-flowing river.

'I'll have you out of the water soon, mate. Don't worry.'

If I didn't get him onto the island there was no way I was going to get him to the shore before he succumbed to the bitter temperature of the water. I paddled as strongly as I was able and headed, as best I could with my additional load, towards the small shingle beach which formed the top of the island. At the point where I thought we were going to make it, in the final few yards, the current kicked in and spun us around and off the headland, pushing us back into the main flow of the river.

I paddled for all I was worth to counter this and drive us back towards the island before we were swept past it. At first it seemed like a losing battle, but then miraculously we caught an eddy that helpfully spun us towards a relatively gentle patch of water by the shoreline. It provided us with some very welcome respite from the fierce flow of current rushing by, enough for me to paddle us both onto the beach. I felt the hull of my kayak slide reassuringly to a stop on the shingle and breathed a huge sigh of relief.

My friend in the water let go of my boat and pulled himself a couple of yards up the beach, dragging his boat with him to prevent it being washed away. Then he collapsed, half in and half out of the icy water and simply lay there.

'You can't stay there, mate,' I shouted. 'You'll freeze to death.' I extricated myself from my cockpit and stepped ashore, dragging my boat safely onto the low-lying island before helping him to his feet and leading him up onto a low grassy bank just clear of the shoreline.

I encouraged him to walk about and warm himself up, while I grabbed my spare emergency clothing out of my kayak. Although we'd managed to salvage his boat, it seemed he'd lost all of his spare kit. I started up my gas camping stove and boiled up water for tea, the solution to all of life's problems. Then I helped him change out of his wet clothes and into my dry ones. By the time the tea was ready he was warmer and a little more talkative. A couple of the other competitors paddled by, travelling so fast in the current it was all I could do to shout briefly what had happened and ask them to send help before they were gone. Even then I wasn't sure they'd understood.

'I can't believe I've lost my new carbon-fibre paddle,' my new friend murmured miserably.

'Sorry?'

'I paid $400 for a brand-new carbon fibre paddle. It snapped when I went over, I won't be seeing that again.'

I had hoped I might have inadvertently rescued a dot-com millionaire; it would have helped with the sponsorship money. But I suspected now I might be out of luck.

My cries to the passing racers must have been understood, because an hour or so later a small speedboat powered back up the river towards us. The two race volunteers on board, part of a fantastic group of people who make the race possible each year, collected my now reheated and dry friend. They dragged his kayak across their boat, inverted and at right angles (it looked like they'd done this before). After some warm-spirited handshakes and thanks, the three of them disappeared back up the river, presumably to the next checkpoint with access to a road.

I now found myself alone, and once more engulfed by that eerie Yukon twilight on a tiny island in the middle of a vast Canadian wilderness. My only spare clothing was now making its way up the river on my new friend and I was down at least four teabags. To make matters worse, I now had an unexpected extra couple of hours to make up on the rest of the racers. I slipped back into my kayak and pushed off into the rapidly flowing river. I figured I'd better get a move on.

* * *

Later that day, paddling steadily along a wider, slower stretch of the river, an unusual shape in the water caught my eye. I paddled over, reached down and pulled it out. I laughed out loud. It was my new friend's carbon fibre paddle. He was right, it had snapped but it was still in one piece, the carbon fibre weave holding the two broken sections together at the break. It was repairable. That'll cheer him up, I thought, and stowed it behind me in the cargo net on the back of my kayak. I'd get it back to him at the end of the race.

Further along the route I pulled over at a checkpoint station. As I stepped out of my boat and made my way up the bank, I noticed a familiar figure in front of me already enjoying the hospitality of the check point. It was Riggs. I was amazed I'd managed to catch up with him and pleasantly surprised to find I wouldn't be paddling the rest of the race on my own after all.

'How are you doing, mate?' I asked.

'Bloody hell,' he said smiling, 'they've just been telling me what happened to you. I was wondering where you'd disappeared to. One of the other teams said you'd capsized and were stuck on an island somewhere.'

He pushed a steaming hot mug in my direction. 'Cup of tea, mate?'

Over the years on my ocean rowing adventures, I'd spent countless shifts rowing alone on deck at night. The combination of exhaustion and lack of sleep inevitably led to hallucinations from time to time. It's almost an occupational hazard on an ocean rowing boat. Never, though, not once, have I hallucinated as vividly or as terrifyingly as during the later stages of the Yukon River race.

Riggs and I were easing into our second full night on the water. We'd completed a compulsory stop a little earlier in the day at

Carmacks, a small campsite situated on the Yukon. We'd been able to grab a few hours' sleep there and a welcome burger before setting off once again. Even with the rest stop, fatigue and lack of sleep were increasingly becoming an issue. The unnerving night-time twilight of the Yukon in June only served to add to our disorientation and exhaustion.

'There are lights on the water coming towards me, Riggs, can you see them?' I shouted at him across the water between us. 'They're floating candles, hundreds of them!' I said, alarmed. Even now I can recall the sight vividly and the anxiety it instilled in me.

Riggs, fighting his own personal battle with fatigue, had little in the way of explanation. 'There's nothing there, mate,' he said wearily. 'You're seeing things.'

It got worse. The candles became posters floating on the surface of the river surrounding my boat. They were posters and the front pages of newspapers, all with what appeared to be missing persons photographs on them.

Then, as I looked towards the bank in that horrible half-light, the trees seemed to morph into the shape of what appeared to be members of some old pioneer family. Grown men, women and children, all dressed like they'd emerged from a John Ford Western, were urging me to come towards them. It was incredibly disturbing and faintly sinister, but utterly convincing.

'I can see people on the bank calling us over,' I shouted to Riggs. 'Can you see them?'

'Mate, there's nothing there. You're imagining it.'

This went on for the best part of an hour. It wasn't like falling asleep and having a vivid dream where you think you're awake when you're not. That had often happened on my ocean rowing adventures. This was like being transported to another reality. I was wide awake. I had to be to keep the kayak upright, but nothing I could see was real, nothing I could see was there. I was aware of this but still found myself unable to do anything about it. I was completely at the mercy of these intense hallucinations. My exhausted, sleep-starved and no doubt dehydrated brain was transporting me into my own personal horror film, seemingly created from subconscious fears this vast wilderness instilled in me.

'Oh fuck!' I said, becoming angry and finally running out of patience with myself. 'Now I'm seeing bears!'

I was paddling closer to the shore and a large patch of shallowing shingle. In front of me, there appeared to be four black bears standing motionless in the water, ten yards out into the river, staring intently in my direction as I approached.

'I can see four bears now, standing right in front of me!' I shouted to Riggs.

'Mick!' Riggs shouted over from the middle of the river. 'They're real bears!'

A burst of adrenalin rocketed into my bloodstream and I started paddling ferociously to get away from the bank where the four very real bears were waiting. My sudden and urgent reaction to Riggs's warning had a similar effect on the bears. They bolted like startled dogs, fortunately in the opposite direction, disappearing into the surrounding woods. I paddled away relieved and now very much clear-headed, out towards Riggs in the middle of the river. He was still laughing uncontrollably when I reached him.

Meanwhile, up ahead, Steve and Si had separated. Si had pushed on, looking for a top-three finish, and Steve had partnered up with a veteran Yukon paddler called Gary. Gary had helpfully offered to swap Steve's bulky rental paddle for his more lightweight and user-friendly spare. Steve also found him a mine of useful tips on coping with the race as it reached its critical later stages.

Gary explained to Steve how in one of his previous Yukon races he'd become trapped in fast-flowing shallow water beneath a fallen tree. He'd been terrified that he would drown before somehow managing to drag himself free. It had left him shaken and the psychological scars apparently were still evident.

As their final night on the river closed in around him, Gary was struggling to keep going. Exhausted, like everyone else battling the lack of sleep, the worry of being trapped again was becoming a debilitating fear: he might not be so lucky next time. He wanted to stop, to pull out of the race. Steve, to his credit, talked him around and kept him going through this low point. He even took over navigating responsibilities while Gary got through his period of self-doubt and exhaustion.

Steve Grenham on the Yukon River was a far cry from the Steve Grenham whose door I knocked on early one Saturday morning for our first training run on the River Ouse, little more than six months previously.

I was having my own mental battle in the latter stages of the race. The hallucinations were still plaguing me from time to time and I was increasingly exhausted. My kayak, designed for paddling in rough water, was shorter than Riggs's and consequently had a slower hull speed. I was paddling furiously most of the time simply to keep up with him. My rehydration and rest routine, which had served me well when paddling alone, fell apart. I became increasingly dehydrated and frustrated. It was like going for a run with someone when you're wearing boots and they're wearing running shoes.

I was becoming increasingly bad tempered and irritable, but instead of simply explaining to Riggs and asking for him to slow down while I got myself together, I tried to battle through it. I wasn't used to being the weak link and I wasn't dealing with it well. Annoyingly, I was well aware of what was happening but seemingly unable to prevent myself from making all the wrong decisions. It was like watching myself hurtle towards a car crash.

Riggs bit his tongue and put up with my erratic mood swings and rambling gibberish through the whole episode. To make matters worse, early in the morning the next day we then found ourselves caught in a fierce storm with torrential rain and head-on gale-force winds. Even with the formidable Yukon River current in our favour, our speed was reduced dramatically, and we were reduced to paddling within feet of the shoreline to try to gain some small level of protection.

Perversely, the downturn in the weather seemed to help my situation. By the time we'd battled out of the storm we were near a check station at Fort Selkirk where there was food and drink on offer, not to mention a toilet. We stopped to have a drink and a short rest and, by the time we left, I was pretty much back on track again. Looking back, I suspect I may have been close to collapse, as I'd foolishly allowed myself to become needlessly dehydrated and everything else had sprung from that. Fortunately, my paddling partner had been a good enough friend to put up with it and get me through it. Once more I was in his debt.

Seventy hours after we began, Riggs and I paddled into Dawson City. Si and Steve had already arrived safely, well ahead of us. They both cheered us in along the last stretch of the river and helped us wearily out of our boats. The whole of the Cockleshell Endeavour team had successfully completed one of the toughest kayak races in the world. It had been an incredible experience, as fantastic as it had been difficult.

The Impact on Steve was obvious. He'd come in ninth in the solo kayak class. His increasing self-respect and growing self-esteem were evident. The kayaking had been incredible but, even better than that, the Cockleshell Endeavour was working. Steve was rapidly getting back on track.

CHAPTER 12

HARSH REALITY

The Yukon, like the Great Glen and Devizes expeditions before it, had been a great success. However, neither Steve Grenham nor I were anywhere near the level we needed to be as solo kayakers to realistically attempt a circumnavigation of the Falklands. We'd made massive strides in an incredibly short space of time, but kayaking in land waterways, even ones as demanding as the Yukon, did not equate to paddling around the Falkland Islands at the mercy of the Southern Ocean.

If we were to complete our original goal, we needed to shift the focus and intensity of our training. We needed to get offshore and train in conditions as similar as possible to those we might expect to find in the southern hemisphere. I knew absolutely the risks and dangers which lay ahead and what we needed to prepare for.

I contacted the legendary international paddler and kayak designer Nigel Dennis for advice. He offered to provide a pair of kayaks for us to trial and recommended a training school which could help with our ongoing training. A few weeks later, in early September, Steve and I were en route to a ten-day training camp on the Isle of Man. The plan was to complete a week's training and then to finish our stay with a three-day circumnavigation of the island.

The training week was invaluable, both in terms of tuition and experience on the open water. The weather proved testing and unpredictable. We had balmy windless blue skies to work under one moment only to see raging gales the next. The weather combined with the Irish Sea and the formidable island coastline to create an excellent if sometimes daunting training ground.

Despite our undoubted progress, one thing was becoming increasingly clear: Steve's confidence offshore was nothing like as strong as it was during the races and expeditions we'd previously embarked upon.

Stepping back onto the sea felt like going home to me. I wasn't intimidated by the conditions and the environment. My kayaking skills may have been limited but my rowing and sailing history left me completely at home on the sea. I respected it but, crucially, I could assess the situations and understand what was happening and why. It was an almost completely new experience for Steve and as such a far more daunting one. I could see he was operating well out of his comfort zone at times. One training camp was not going to alter that.

With the weather forecast predicting increasingly strong north-westerly winds, a successful circumnavigation of the island in the last three days of our stay looked unlikely. We decided instead to extend our training by a day or two before embarking on couple of days' distance paddling on our own along the more sheltered east coast. Those trips would prove to be the final confirmation, if it were needed, that we were not ready to venture out on the Southern Ocean.

With just the two of us on the water, Steve soon slipped back into the 'go for it' attitude that had become apparent on the Great Glen expedition. That might have been less of an issue if he hadn't been so fast in a straight line, or I had been a more proficient paddler. As it was, it made difficult situations potentially lethal. At one point, crossing a large bay with the wind picking up, my rudder chose just that moment to fail. A line snapped and I found myself struggling to maintain direction against the building wind and waves. I shouted out to Steve for help but it was too late – he was already disappearing into the distance, aiming for the next headland. I made a course for the nearest stretch of beach to repair my boat while Steve journeyed alone across the bay. We eventually met up an hour or so later, a few miles along the beach.

It was clear, with the best will in the world, that operating as a team in solo boats we were a disaster waiting to happen. It was another sobering lesson for me of the consequences if a similar situation developed paddling the wild, freezing and unpredictable waters surrounding the Falklands. A repetition would potentially prove fatal for one or both of us. I didn't possess the kayaking skills to bolster Steve's confidence and to allow us to operate effectively as a team. What was worse, I could see Steve's confidence wilting under the pressure of being offshore in these increasingly challenging conditions. He was no longer enjoying the experience; he was enduring it. It was becoming counterproductive. There was simply no way we were equipped, individually or as a team, to make a successful circumnavigation of the Falkland Islands. That realisation came with a dreadful sense of failure. I felt stumbling at this last hurdle tarnished everything we'd already achieved.

I had to remind myself, yet again, that this wasn't about the kayaking goals – it was about Steve making positive steps towards recovery. We didn't fail if we didn't meet the kayaking goals. We failed if we didn't keep Steve's recovery on track. If I could keep that going, improve on the undoubted results we'd already achieved, we could still build on the project's success. I just needed to find a way to do that.

At the end of our time training around the Isle of Man, it was apparent to both of us that our planned return to the Falklands in little more than three months, the following January, was not feasible. It had to be then in order to take advantage of the southern hemisphere summer, and it was just too soon. It was an easy and obvious decision to make and I think a relief to Steve. I still had no doubt that, given time, we were more than capable of reaching the standard required, but we simply had no way of putting that time and training in place before the start date.

We would have to become full-time kayakers for at least three months of continued paddling and tuition in advance of any return to the Falklands. There was no way we could finance such a commitment, even if we could find the time. We both agreed we'd have to postpone any return to the islands until we had put that training in place and were properly prepared. It was a disappointment, but it wasn't the end of the road, just a setback. We hoped.

With the postponement of our return to the Falkland Islands, I disappeared to a new job in America skippering a private yacht for a retired American couple. Steve returned to the construction contract he was working on in Brighton. Despite our positive intentions, there was every possibility that the Cockleshell Endeavour project could have faded away and died at that point. Steve had already gained a lot from the experience; he was fit and healthy again. His self-confidence had been restored and, most importantly, he was communicating with people. He was talking about his issues and people, primarily his family, were listening to him. I remember asking him once after a day's winter training on the River Ouse, in the run up to the Isle of Man trip: 'Is this kayaking making a difference for you, mate?'

'Well, I'm talking to Aicha now about stuff I never would have spoken about before. Just the fact that I'm prepared to speak about PTSD with her is an improvement. It's helping me, and, more importantly, it's helping her. It's been much tougher for her and my family than me,' he replied.

Many of our kayaking trips and almost all our training had involved working together as a pair in a small boat over long hours, so naturally we'd talked a lot. It helped that we were both former marines, that we had a shared history and that, basically, we both spoke the same language. It was a key theme of the Cockleshell Endeavour as far as I was concerned. Put two guys together who have that shared background, give them a challenge to rise to and the rest will fall into place. They'll work together to overcome that problem and, in doing so, as a natural consequence, they'll talk about other things. It will help break down the isolation many people can feel when suffering with a physical or mental health issue.

Physical challenges, by definition, improve mental and physical fitness, which naturally impacts positively on mental health recovery, particularly depression. Striving for and achieving goals creates self-confidence, instils belief and boosts self-esteem in an individual. These factors were the natural by-products of our kayak training, let alone the races and expeditions we completed. In less than a year the difference in Steve's demeanour and personality was clear to everyone who knew him.

In truth, we'd already achieved what we'd set out to achieve. Steve was well and truly back on the road to recovery. The Cockleshell Endeavour project had undoubtedly been a success, regardless of any return to the Falkland Islands. Still, it didn't sit well with me that we hadn't made it back to the islands as we'd originally promised. It felt like there was unfinished business.

When we moved away from the two-man kayaks for the expeditions, Steve had become isolated again – we all had. It became more about achieving a kayaking goal individually than the benefits of working in close proximity with a teammate towards achieving that goal. Worst of all, the opportunity to talk as easily as we could in a pairs boat was lost.

On the Great Glen and the training runs off the Isle of Man, by virtue of paddling in one-man boats, we'd spoken less, and we'd become more easily isolated, both completely engrossed in overcoming our own individual challenges. Particularly when the conditions deteriorated, and we were working to the limits of, or perhaps beyond, our abilities. Those challenges were all the more consuming and isolating due to our limited ability to deal with them.

It occurred to me, while transiting the Panama Canal some months later, that returning to the Falklands in a pairs boat might bring that elusive final goal within our grasp. If we looked at using a two-man folding kayak and adjusted our aim from a complete circumnavigation of the whole of the Falkland Islands, a distance of well over 600 miles, to a reduced paddle around East Falkland, a more manageable 120 miles or so, our challenge would become more achievable. It would also hold more relevance. We'd be able to tour many of the significant battle sites of the war in 1982 and, with a little planning, we could also involve the local community. Paddling a folding kayak would require less in terms of technical ability. I had the navigational knowledge, the seagoing experience, and a reduced distance in a more stable boat would not require the months of training that an attempt in one-man kayaks would. We could achieve our goal and end the project on the perfect note.

I contacted Steve from the US to let him know what I'd been thinking. We'd be a year later than planned, simply because we'd missed our summer weather window, and we'd have to make a few adjustments to the original plan, but we could return to the Falkland Islands to make good on our promise. And it would be 2017 – the thirty-fifth anniversary of the Falklands War.

Steve liked the idea. The Cockleshell Endeavour would continue for one more adventure.

CHAPTER 13

THE SUN ALWAYS SHINES ON THE RIGHTEOUS

I finished my contract in the States and headed back to the UK for some final training and preparation ahead of our southern hemisphere adventure, with Steve and I eventually returning to the Falklands in March 2017. But our training partners, Riggs and Si Reed, weren't able to join us. As before, our status as veterans of the war in 1982 meant we were eligible for heavily subsidised flights to and from the islands, which made the whole project financially viable; our teammates, sadly, were not.

Our plan was to paddle from the landing sites of the 1982 conflict at San Carlos, around East Falkland via Darwin and Goose Green, and back along the coast into the capital, Stanley, a journey of around 120 miles. The first order of the day was to make it work logistically.

It would be relatively easy to get myself and Steve down to the Falklands again, but getting our kayak and equipment to the islands was not as simple. Fortunately, we had contacts in the islands who were eager to help. Gary Clement, our driver to Surf Bay on our initial visit, was a former Royal Marine who'd served on a year-long detachment in the Falklands before the war as well as taking part in the liberation. He was now resident there and keen to help. He proved to be invaluable in the planning of our kayaking expedition. Gary put me in touch with people in the military garrison who could potentially help with our transportation issues.

Fergie Clift, a Royal Air Force warrant officer, and Royal Navy Lieutenant Commander Rocky Hudson enthusiastically adopted the project. Although unable to offer guarantees, as operational requirements would always come first, they assured us there was every chance they would be able to transport the equipment down for us ahead of our arrival. It meant thinning the kit list down to the bare minimum to keep the weight down, but it would be possible.

Fergie, who was a keen paddler himself, assured us he had or could find most of the equipment and stores we'd need locally, so we wouldn't need to transport everything with the kayak. Once again, that central theme which seemed to run through all our projects came to the fore just when we needed it most. People who'd never met us, when they heard what we were trying to do, always asked: 'How can we help?' It was humbling and made everything we achieved possible.

Liberty Lodge was fully occupied when Steve and I returned in March 2017. It didn't matter. As Gary Clement had already pointed out, there was no problem finding beds for us in the local community for our stay either side of the expedition. More than that, when word spread of what we were attempting to do, which it did rapidly in such a close-knit community, there were people offering to put us up at every stop on the journey. Initially we'd assumed we would be under canvas every night. As it turned out, even in the most remote areas of the island there were locals who were offering us food and a roof over our heads.

We were both more than familiar with the extremes of weather we'd be facing during our paddle around East Falkland, so we gratefully accepted the offers of hospitality. The last night before Stanley would be spent under canvas, however, as we felt we had to spend at least one night beneath the stars at the mercy of the elements to justify our efforts.

Our hosts in Stanley before we set off were Terrence and Carol Philips, typically warm and hospitable Falkland Islanders.

We couldn't have been made more welcome. Another former marine who's now resident in the islands, Mick 'Pinky' Floyd, was hosting our support team: Marty Gear and Ric Strange. Marty and Ric had served alongside Pinky during the war in the same section.

We would begin the expedition from Port San Carlos, the scene of the initial British landings, when the task force arrived to liberate the islands in May 1982. John and Michelle Jones, who own the farm there, put us up for the night and provided a hearty breakfast before departure.

Marty Gear had been one of my instructors during my Royal Marines basic training, and he and Ric were in Air Defence Troop with me when we landed in 1982. It was as significant a trip for them as it was for Steve and me, if not more so, as they'd both been involved in some of the heaviest fighting during the war.

On 17 March 2017, we hastily unfurled our folding kayak on a tiny beach at the western edge of the settlement. With the breeze picking up, we pushed off to cross the San Carlos River and paddle around the headland opposite and along to San Carlos settlement, our first planned stop. This would take us into San Carlos Water, better known as Bomb Alley during the conflict, thanks to the repeated number of Argentine air attacks on the task force anchored there.

We were in drysuits and fully equipped for cold and wet conditions. Within minutes of waving goodbye to our cheering supporters on the beach, and just a few hundred yards offshore, the Falklands weather welcomed us.

The breezy gusts increased in strength, and minutes later the waves rose up in sympathy. Our course ran almost directly across the wind, heading diagonally for the other side of the wide river. This left us almost beam on to the waves. Even in the sturdy

Wayland kayak we were using for the expedition, it felt vulnerable. To make matters worse, as we were powering through the increasingly difficult conditions, our rudder jammed. I couldn't steer the boat.

The storm was continuing to pick up, as were the accompanying waves it generated. The wind was bitterly cold and the water freezing. Only minutes into our expedition it felt like we were a million miles away from the cosy farmhouse where we'd only recently enjoyed breakfast.

'The rudder's jammed,' I shouted back to Steve.

'Oh shit! We're well fucked then!' Steve shouted. 'We need to get to that beach!' Instantly he began paddling frantically behind me.

I was shocked. It was a problem but not an emergency. We could steer the boat with our paddles until we could get ashore to fix the rudder. His reaction had taken me by surprise. It was a problem at an awkward time but one that was easily remedied. It occurred to me that this was exactly the sort of situation where, if we'd been in separate boats, he'd have paddled away, head down, towards the next piece of dry land.

I shouted back at him over the wind that we were fine, it was nothing we couldn't sort. I asked him to raise the rudder out of the water; the control line was next to him at the back of the boat. That would enable us to steer a course simply by paddling. As soon as the rudder was lifted clear of the water we easily regained control of our direction, problem solved. Steve settled down. The crisis was over.

It was clear to me why Steve had reacted in such an aggressive way to the situations we'd encountered paddling solo on our earlier trips. It was an instinctive reaction, somewhere between fight and flight – an automatic response to an unfamiliar and potentially dangerous situation. In solo kayaks difficult situations could soon develop into potentially lethal ones. In a tandem kayak the problem was resolved in a matter of seconds, working together as a team. It had been the right decision to go back to a two-man boat.

The rest of the day passed uneventfully. We fixed the rudder at a beach further along the route and reached San Carlos settlement by early afternoon. After the excitement at the start of the paddle, it proved ultimately to be a relatively gentle introduction to the expedition, with the squall disappearing just as swiftly as it had arrived.

San Carlos Settlement was the place where all four of us had stepped ashore in 1982 along with many of the British troops. It seemed to have changed little in the three-and-a-half decades since. With one exception: the cemetery which stands as a memorial to all of the 255 British servicemen killed in the conflict and the final resting place for 13 of them. Shaped like a circular stone sheep corral, it stands on the forwards slope of the settlement overlooking San Carlos Water. It's a fitting monument to those who didn't return and a sombre reminder to those of us who did how fortunate we were.

My old friend Jonathan Scott had tragically passed away after a valiant battle against cancer in June 2015, leaving behind a devastated widow and young family. He'd landed with 40 Commando at Port San Carlos in 1982. I'd asked his wife Kate and their children if there was something of his we could take to leave as a memorial. They eventually decided on a training shoe. He was a keen runner throughout his life, completing marathons to raise money for charity until the later stages of his cruel illness. They thought he'd like the idea. They included a waterproofed letter of explanation to be buried with it.

The four of us found a suitable piece of high ground to the north of the cemetery. We dug a hole and, after a few words to remember Scotty, buried the memento that would ensure he would always remain a small part of the Falkland Islands.

Early the following morning we pushed off from the beach at the settlement to make our way back up San Carlos Water. It was a very early start and pitch black. We were paddling towards the headland, Chancho Point, and out into the channel between East and West Falkland, Falkland Sound. Our early departure was to ensure we rounded the headland before the stronger winds arrived later in the day.

It was still and almost windless as we pushed off into the intimidating darkness. The surrounding land and water merged into one blurred and inky backdrop. Just a few distant stars were visible to help orientate us as we paddled steadily towards the mouth of San Carlos Water.

Many ships were hit in Bomb Alley during the early part of the war in 1982. Including the one I was waiting to disembark from, the troop landing ship RFA *Sir Lancelot*. Fortunately, the 1000-lb bomb which hit us failed to detonate and we were able to safely abandon ship. This was a common occurrence in the early days of the landings: many ships had been hit but the bombs had mercifully failed to detonate, which was due to the high speeds and low altitude the aircraft were flying at to avoid being shot down. The bombs simply didn't have time to fuse before hitting their targets.

HMS *Antelope*, a type 21 frigate protecting the entrance to San Carlos Water, was one of these ships. An attack by four A-4 Skyhawks left her with one crew member killed and two unexploded 1000-lb bombs lodged inside her. She limped into the shallow waters off Ajax Bay in San Carlos Water to anchor while engineers attempted to defuse the bombs. One of the bombs detonated during the process, killing one member of the bomb disposal team and badly injuring the other. The explosion ripped a hole in *Antelope*'s hull from the water line to the funnel. The resulting fires raging on board forced the captain to issue the order to abandon ship. He was the last man to leave.

Five minutes later, the missile magazines ignited, breaking *Antelope*'s back in a spectacular explosion. The dying warship was silhouetted against the night sky by the blast, becoming one of the iconic images of the war. She remained defiantly afloat the next day but was broken in two. The crippled and smoking remnants of the ship slowly disappeared beneath the surface of the water. My ship, which would be hit later that morning in another air attack, was anchored next to *Antelope*. I had watched it all unfold.

Antelope remains in Falkland Sound, her final resting place marked by a buoy which stands guard directly above her broken hull. In the shallow waters she could easily become a hazard to navigation. I had hoped that we would be able to see the buoy as we paddled back out of San Carlos Water, but knew there was no chance of that in the darkness which engulfed us.

So it came as quite a shock when emerging from the darkness sometime later that a huge shape loomed over us. No lights, just the intimidating black silhouette of the buoy marking *Antelope*'s final resting place. The fact that we'd paddled right up to it by chance was incredible.

We stopped for a moment. Apparently in daylight the pristine waters allow for a clear view of the ship just a few yards below. In the darkness we could see nothing. Royal Navy divers regularly replace the ship's ensign, or flag, which still flies from her stern mast. It was an eerie thought that only a few feet beneath us her ensign was still proudly flying after thirty-five years, only now moving to the flow of the icy waters which consumed her.

We left *Antelope* and her solitary marker behind and rounded the headland at the entrance to Bomb Alley. We paddled out into the more exposed waters of Falkland Sound just as dawn broke.

Two days later we arrived at Darwin and Goose Green, where our support team, Ric and Marty, were there to greet us. It was a location which had great significance for them, as they'd both fought in the battle of Goose Green, providing air defence for the parachute regiment. Ric had been mentioned in dispatches after standing up during the battle to shoot down an Argentine plane attacking the advancing British forces.

One of our sponsors, Kev Browning, MD of Global Tunnelling Experts, had been held prisoner at Goose Green throughout the occupation. Kev, along with 113 other members of the local community, was placed under armed guard for twenty-nine days in the tiny village hall. They would be in the middle of the battle that raged over two days as 2 PARA fought to liberate them. He was a teenager growing up in the islands when the Argentines invaded; immediately after the liberation he travelled to the UK and enlisted in the Parachute Regiment.

We intended staying overnight and pushing off the following morning. The weather had other ideas. Gales descended, and we settled in for an unplanned extra day in Goose Green. It proved a fortunate delay, allowing Marty and Ric more time to reflect on their experiences thirty-five years earlier. They walked Steve and me through the battle. It was fascinating to see the way both men recalled the experience in different ways. Marty remembered specific episodes in detail, even down to the smell of burning gorse in the later stages of the battle, but there were large parts he'd simply forgotten. Ric, on the other hand, appeared to have an almost photographic recall of events, at one time even locating the remnants of an enemy trench which had pinned the paras down during their advance. He confided in me at one point that the experience was, in his own words, 'On a constant loop in my head.'

The wreckage of the Aermacchi aircraft Ric shot down was amazingly still strewn around the area. Remarkably, Ric had been tracked down via social media a few years earlier. The pilot's brother wanted to speak to Ric, he wanted to know how his sibling had died. Although the pilot was identified and his remains buried on the island, the Argentine government had never officially admitted his death. He was still supposedly missing in action. Unforgivably, the pilot's mother had gone to her grave expecting her son one day to walk through the door again. It was a wicked and unnecessary added cruelty. His brother wanted closure for himself and his family. He couldn't get that from the Argentine authorities, so he had tracked down Ric to try to learn the full details of his brother's death. It was a tough conversation for both parties but ultimately a positive one. With the help of Ric's information the Red Cross eventually completed a DNA crossmatch on the pilot's remains. Only a couple of years before our return, the results allowed the pilot, Teniente De Fragata Daniel Enrique Miguel, to be buried in his own marked grave. Three members of his family were able to attend the ceremony on the island. The pilot's sister-in-law contacted Ric to tell him that: 'Although he had taken him away he had also given him back to his family.' It was closure for them and perhaps for Ric, too.

Departing Goose Green a day later than planned, we headed straight along Choiseul Sound towards the port at Mare Harbour. There was a small Royal Naval detachment there who were our hosts for the night. After a good night's rest, we found ourselves waking early to a slap-up full English breakfast prepared by our hosts, two Royal Navy warrant officers. Nothing, it seemed, was too much trouble for our hosts wherever we stopped.

We pushed off from Bertha's Beach that morning into a stiff breeze through breaking waves. Having left the relative protection of Choiseul Sound behind us, we were now transiting the southeast corner of East Falklands. There was nothing to the right of us now other than the vast and ferocious Southern Ocean.

We'd already had a glimpse of the incredible wildlife that thrives on the islands. Seals had playfully investigated us, and on one occasion we came across what appeared to be two young leopard seals basking on a rock. Fortunately, there was no sign of their adult contemporaries. Leopard seals are apex predators, which grow to over twelve feet in length, and there have been accounts of attacks on humans in the past. We'd been warned to avoid three things by the locals before we set off. The first was mine-fields and the second, leopard seals.

Heading out from Bertha's Beach we had to round Elephant Island, named after the huge colony of elephant seals that occupy it. We could smell and hear the enormous animals before we could see them. We gave the island a wide enough berth so as not to alarm them, but close enough to afford us a glimpse of these spectacular creatures. Paddling near these fabulous animals, as elegant in the water as they are ungainly out of it, was a once-in-a-lifetime experience. We were beginning to see the islands in a very different way.

We also began to experience another less welcome characteristic of the Falkland Islands, the third thing we were advised to avoid: kelp. There are miles and miles of kelp beds along the south-east coastline. Where possible we avoided it. When we couldn't, it became a soul-destroying, painfully slow process to drag ourselves through it, the kelp cloying at the hull of the kayak and entangling our paddles on every stroke. It was impossible to develop a rhythm and every yard gained became an exhausting effort.

Despite this unwanted, if not unexpected, setback, by late afternoon we eventually made it to our next port of call, Fitzroy, near Bluff Cove. It would be our last stop before a night under canvas and our final day's paddle to the finish in Stanley.

Fitzroy and Bluff Cove saw the biggest single loss of life for British forces during the war. The troop landing ships *Sir Galahad* and *Sir Tristram* were both hit in an air raid, killing forty-eight men on board *Galahad* and two on *Tristram*. *Sir Galahad*, beyond repair, was eventually scuttled and is now a designated war grave. A Royal Marine landing craft, *Foxtrot 4*, from HMS *Fearless*, was also attacked and sunk with the loss of six crew in Choiseul Sound. It happened during the same series of attacks, as the vessel made its way to Bluff Cove; four Royal Marines and two naval ratings were lost.

It was a sombre experience to paddle into a stretch of water with such a violent and tragic history, not least for me, as I'd been turned away from boarding the *Galahad* just prior to the attack which sank her. Our experiences with the elephant seals and the struggles through the kelp beds paled into insignificance in comparison.

A warm bed and an equally warm welcome once more awaited us as we landed at Fitzroy. Many of the locals who'd come through the war in 1982 took the time to meet us in the local hall. It was fascinating to hear their stories and experiences and the effect the war had, and still has, on them. In 1982 I may have spoken to two or three Falkland Islanders during the conflict, and then only briefly. The best thing about returning in 2017 was the chance to meet so many, listen to their experiences and become great friends with many of them.

The following morning we pushed off on what we hoped would be the penultimate day of our voyage. The weather forecast wasn't great – it was due to close in with stronger winds and rain. We decided to meet our support team at a small bay almost halfway between Fitzroy and the day's final destination, Mullet Creek. We'd then transport the kayak a short distance overland to another longer inland stretch of water which offered us some protection from the full impact of the Southern Ocean.

It would prove to be the toughest day's paddle of the whole trip. Grey skies began to dominate and, crossing an exposed stretch of water early in the day, we were met with strong headwinds. It was cold, wet and miserable work battling the conditions towards the bay.

We'd had incredibly good luck up until then. The notoriously fickle Falkland Islands weather had generally smiled kindly on us. As Steve regularly reminded me: 'The sun always shines on the righteous, Mick.'

Only one day had been lost so far, to the gales in Goose Green. Now, as we fought the increasing headwinds and building waves, we worried that the weather might prevent us paddling into Stanley the next day. Our mood wasn't lifted by the prospect of our planned night under canvas. We couldn't have picked a worse night. It was shaping up for a grim and possibly premature end to our expedition.

By the time we made it safely into the bay to get our short lift to the next protected stretch of water, it had already been a very tough day's paddling. We were little more than halfway to our planned overnight stop and several hours of gruelling paddling lay ahead. We loaded our kayak onto the roof of our support wagon and gratefully took the lift to the next beach a few hundred metres across country.

Several hours later, tired and soaking wet from frequent heavy showers, we entered Mullet Creek, a meandering muddy estuary running inland for a couple of miles. A colony of young albatrosses greeted us with panicked squawks from the bank overlooking the entrance. There were hundreds of them. Bizarrely, they staggered drunkenly down into the water in front of us with wings spread wide in alarm. The next half hour was spent shepherding this huge flock of young birds along the narrowing stretch of water ahead of us, their panicked cries heralding our arrival. Much like the elephant seals the day before, this was a scene you could only hope to see in the Falkland Islands.

We paddled to the end of the creek, where it disappeared to little more than a muddy stream. The albatrosses had long since departed, presumably back to their nesting place at the entrance. Ric and Marty had slowly picked a drivable route across the unforgiving terrain to reach us, and we looked around for a suitably sheltered area to make camp, never easy to find in the Falklands, particularly in bad weather.

Ric had a better idea. 'See those houses up there,' he pointed into the distance. 'Let's go knock on their doors and see if we can pitch our tents in the garden. Hopefully they'll have mercy on us and invite us in for a wet of tea.' He laughed.

We pulled our kayak up onto the bank, rolled it over to prevent it filling with rainwater and jumped in the Land Rover.

There were two houses at the end of a long gravel track. Ric knocked at the door of the first. 'Sorry for bothering you. We're the support team for a couple of vets circumnavigating East Falkland in a kayak. Is there any chance we could put our tents up in your garden tonight?' Ric asked.

The lady who answered the door replied slowly, 'I know exactly who you are and no you can't put your tents up in our garden. You can all come in and stay in the house and I'll cook you a nice steak.'

Our planned night under canvas never materialised. None of us were disappointed. The four of us were warmly welcomed into Stephen and Ann Luxton's home for the last night of our adventure. Their hospitality mirrored perfectly the welcome we'd received since the moment we'd set foot on the islands again.

*   *   *

The following morning we woke to lighter winds and thankfully no rain. The forecast looked promising, but this was the Falklands, where you can experience four seasons in any given day. It was grey and overcast but a vast improvement on the previous day. Crucially, there were no strong winds.

We dragged our kayak for the first mile along the estuary as the floodtide slowly refilled the creek. When the water was finally deep enough, we stepped back into our boat for what we thought would be the last time and paddled out of the creek past our friends the albatrosses for the final leg of our expedition. They seemed less concerned about our departure than they had been about our arrival.

The final leg, potentially the most dangerous, included the most exposed and vulnerable stretch of our journey. We were paddling north-east, hugging the shoreline as closely as we safely could, heading for Cape Pembroke. To our right, once more nothing but the vast expanse of the Southern Ocean. The formidable ocean swell on display even in mercifully light conditions gave a clue as to how treacherous this stretch of coastline would be in bad weather.

The southern ocean, even subdued, was ominously threatening, crashing into and over the jagged rocks which lie along the coastline. Fields of kelp once more regularly conspired to slow our progress. It felt like we were creeping by a slumbering monster, trying not to wake it, as we edged our way along the coast towards Cape Pembroke in the distance.

After many tense hours we finally rounded the cape. Our relief was palpable. We were turning west now, the last stretch towards Stanley's outer harbour and the protection it would afford us. The weather had thankfully improved throughout the day. We were now paddling beneath a bright sun and beautiful blue skies. It appeared we'd managed to pass by the slumbering ocean monster without disturbing it.

'The sun always shines on the righteous,' I said to Steve, laughing as we basked in the warmth of the glorious day.

A small red, civilian aircraft buzzed us a couple of times, low enough to startle some birds sitting on the ocean nearby. The occupants were waving enthusiastically. We weren't sure if it was a coincidence or if they were the advance section of some kind of welcoming party, but it added to the jubilant atmosphere of our last hours on the water.

We entered the outer harbour in mid-afternoon. We found a spot in behind some protective rocks and took a break, grabbing a quick snack and a drink. We noticed after a while several small boats in the distance apparently heading towards us. Steve and Ann, our generous hosts from the previous night, had driven out on their power boat to welcome us. Alongside there was a small sailing yacht with our support team and a group of enthusiastic friends and supporters on board. There was even a drone overhead filming our arrival. It appeared we did indeed have a welcome party.

A pod of dolphins, at least twenty animals strong, decided to join in the fun. Surrounding our boat, they formed an escort as we paddled in, stopping next to us at times and deliberately splashing us with their tails, like misbehaving kids in a water fight. They stayed with us for close to an hour, right up to the inner harbour, before finally disappearing.

'I hope you realise this isn't normal,' I shouted back to Steve as this joyful mayhem took place all around us. 'All the time I've spent at sea I've never seen anything like this before. You couldn't buy this, mate.'

It seemed he may have had a point all along; the sun did indeed shine on the righteous.

It was the most memorable end to what had been an incredible trip.

Steve shouted to me, obviously enjoying the moment. 'That's Harriet up there,' he said, pointing to the mountain he fought on which overlooks Stanley.

'The radio station wants me to go up there tomorrow to do an interview. It's not happening. I'm not going back to that place. This is my memory of the Falklands Islands now.'

There could have been no better ending for the Cockleshell Endeavour.

CHAPTER 14

MEETING SPARKY

If it was an unlikely coincidence bumping into Steve Grenham, it was a miracle how I ever met Steve Sparkes again. What's more, if I'd been shocked how badly Steve Grenham had been let down in 2014, I was horrified when I discovered how the system had abandoned Sparky three decades earlier.

It was September 2017. I was home in the UK preparing to fly out to St Barts in the Caribbean to begin a new skipper's contract. Not for the first time in my life, a hurricane arrived with harsh and unwelcome consequences. It was devastating for those unfortunate souls in the Caribbean directly in its path, but in a far less traumatic way equally damaging for me, several thousand miles away.

An email from my employer informed me that St Barts had been devastated by Hurricane Irma. The luxury hotel that had employed me to take its VIP guests sailing no longer existed. Neither did my job. But I was still a lot better off than people there who had lost everything, some even their lives.

The Cockleshell Endeavour which Steve Grenham and I had undertaken was complete. A lingering legacy of those adventures was the desperate need for me to return to full-time paid employment as soon as possible. I'd gone to the wall financially to make sure the Cockleshell Endeavour was possible. That was manageable with my new job to look forward too, but this sudden and unexpected change of plan had left me in a precarious financial situation.

One afternoon a friend invited me down to The Coach House in Rottingdean – my local pub – to take my mind off matters, grab some lunch and have a chat about alternative possibilities. When I walked in to meet him, the landlord, Darren, was behind the bar chatting on the phone.

He noticed me and waved, then, covering the mouthpiece on the phone, he said, 'All right, Mick. I've got one of your lot on the line.'

'My lot?' I asked curiously. 'Do you mean a bootneck?' (The nickname for a Royal Marine.)

'Yeah.'

'What's his name?'

'Steve Sparkes. Sparky.'

The name was instantly familiar. 'I know a Steve Sparkes,' I responded.

Darren finished his conversation, put the receiver down and then turned to me.

'Well, you'll see him tonight if you come in. He's coming down.'

That evening I found myself walking back towards the distinctive black bay windows which form the front of the Coach House. I'd been looking forwards to seeing Sparky since Darren told me he was visiting the pub. As I approached the building, though, it suddenly dawned on me that I hadn't seen him in thirty-seven years. Would we have anything in common after all these years? Was this such a great idea after all?

More of a concern was that, despite our mutual history in the Royal Marines, we hadn't actually been close friends. In fact, we'd only ever met once before, just a couple of weeks before I joined the marines in July 1980.

I'd travelled to Commando Training Centre at Lympstone in Devon to watch my brother's troop pass out of training. Sparky was 141 Troop's King's Badge man, the most outstanding recruit. He'd become good friends with my brother during the many challenges of Royal Marine training. The night before the passing out parade, my brother, Sparky and a couple of their other mates had come to visit my parents and me in the nearby hotel where we were staying, just to say hi before their big day. It was the first and only time we met, despite in later years occasionally serving in the same unit.

Approaching the pub, I was beginning to worry that perhaps this wasn't such a great idea. That perhaps there would simply be an awkward silence as two now middle-aged men who'd never really known one another attempted to make small talk. Most of all I was worried I wouldn't even recognise him.

I needn't have been concerned. As I walked through the front door, I saw a small group stood close to the bar. Sparky was facing away from me at an angle and wearing what I would soon learn had become his signature flat cap. I recognised him immediately, even with his back partially turned. I walked towards him smiling and interrupted his conversation.

'Mr Sparkes,' I said, touching his elbow.

He stopped mid-sentence and turned towards me, curious. 'Who's that?'

'Mick Dawson, mate. Steve Dawson's brother. Last time we met was the night before your troop pass out. It's been a while.' I laughed.

'Well, bloody hell. How are you doing, mate?' His face broke into what I now know to be its regular broad smile.

That smile was infectious and ice breaking. I grinned back. Any anxiety over our meeting dissolving in a moment. It was as if the first time we'd met, almost four decades ago, had been just the previous week. The connection with my brother and our shared Royal Marine history broke down any barriers. Anyone looking in on our conversation who didn't know us would have thought it was just two very close mates catching up for the first time after many years, nothing having changed despite the passage of time. In some respects that was indeed the case, except that one thing had changed. As we fell into our easy conversation, I noticed the folded white cane he grasped in his left hand and remembered Sparky was now blind.

CHAPTER 15

SPARKY'S STORY

Steve Sparkes had excelled in Royal Marines training, setting record times on the commando assault courses which had stood for years afterwards.

The endurance course is a brutal two-mile assault course run in full fighting gear and weapons over the gorse-filled, undulating and exhausting terrain of Woodbury Common in Devon. Its route cuts a path through a number of formidable obstacles: neck-high freezing ponds; muddy, energy-sapping bogs; and claustro-phobic tunnels you have to crawl through on your hands and knees and in one, the aptly named Smarty Tube, on your belly. It finishes with a four-mile run back to camp and a live weapons test on the range. A maximum completion time of sixty-four minutes only adds to the pressure. It's one of a series of exhausting physical challenges run on consecutive days which form the commando tests at the end of training. Every Royal Marine must pass these tests to be awarded his green beret.

The records Sparky set in 1980 not only on the endurance course but on the other assault courses in the commando tests, were only bettered when the equipment marines wore was modernised. Sparky was a one-off, an exceptional Royal Marine destined for a stellar career in the corps.

When the Falklands War broke out in 1982, Sparky was a member of K Company 42 Commando, coincidentally the same unit (although not the same company) as Steve Grenham. Sparky formed part of a four-man patrol which for three nights made a series of incredibly dangerous reconnaissance missions into the minefields around the base of the heavily defended Mount Harriet. Their orders were to locate a route through those minefields for the main attack which was to follow.

On the third night, a member of the fire support team who was sent to cover their withdrawal in the event of discovery stepped on a mine. His leg was blown off below the knee and their cover was now compromised. Sparky hoisted the marine onto his shoulder and, with his three remaining comrades crawling ahead on their bellies prodding the ground with bayonets, they painstakingly navigated their way back out of the minefield. Sparky and the rest of the patrol carried the marine for over a mile to the nearest safe landing zone where a helicopter was able to recover him.

Sparky handed the injured man over personally to Dr Rick Jolly, the legendary military surgeon who set up the famous field hospital in Ajax Bay where the British forces landed. This medical centre came to be known as the Red and Green Life Machine – a salute to the beret colours of the Royal Marines and Paratroopers who formed the vast majority of the first troops to land. The proud legacy of Rick Jolly and his incredible team of doctors, nurses and medics is the lifesaving treatment they provided for combatants on both sides of the conflict.

During the subsequent attack on Mount Harriet, Sparky achieved another rare distinction. He became the first British soldier since World War II to be promoted in the field, being made up to corporal after his section commander was shot and killed during the battle. The exceptional promise he'd shown throughout training had continued in the white heat of battle.

On his return from the Falklands, with his star very much on the ascent, he was unsurprisingly immediately selected for promotion and offered a junior command course, an intensive leadership course which was the prerequisite to becoming a fully fledged corporal. In a relatively short space of time, this would have led to his field promotion becoming his permanent rank. He passed that course as always with flying colours.

He would, however, never take the next step on that ladder, let alone reach the very top of it. Life was about to take a catastrophic change of direction for Sparky.

Having passed his Junior Command course and with his career path now on a seemingly relentlessly upward trajectory, Sparky was encouraged to put himself forwards for selection for the Special Boat Service. The SBS is the Royal Marines amphibious equivalent to the Special Air Service, the elite amphibious experts within the British special forces. Sparky's obvious abilities and his conduct during the Falklands War convinced many of his superiors that his future lay at the very pinnacle of soldiering. He decided to try for selection.

As with seemingly everything he put his mind to, Sparky came through that notoriously unforgiving selection process successfully. As a result, he was accepted for training to become one of the world's truly elite soldiers, a swimmer canoeist (SC3).

But just at the point when his future had never looked brighter, tragedy struck.

Towards the end of the incredibly arduous selection process there was a diving exercise using rebreather apparatus. This is a sealed breathing unit, purifying and recycling the air so as not to produce bubbles which could give the divers presence away during covert underwater operations. Sparky and the other potential SC3 candidates were sent down for an extended period of time using this kit, the aim being to familiarise themselves with the equipment but equally as importantly build up the practice hours required to qualify them to use it.

The exercise was at night in murky sea water with almost zero visibility. The aim was for the divers to descend to the seabed (which wasn't particularly deep), find a guide wire that formed a large circular track and follow it. They had to complete a lengthy stay beneath the surface, pulling themselves around this circuit, increasing their familiarity with the specialist equipment they were using. Sparky, unusually, soon found himself struggling.

'At first,' he explained that evening in The Coach House, 'I started to get this really bad headache. I didn't think too much about it and just tried to battle through. It got worse and worse, though, right at the front of my skull. I'd never known pain like it. Then I started to get chest pains and couldn't breathe. I had no choice but to resurface.

'The instructors thought I'd panicked in the darkness and just needed to calm down and sort myself out, so told me to fin to the side and get myself together. Which I did. Then they sent me down again.'

Sparky was the first diver to have problems that night and resurface, but not the last. As he submerged for a second stint around the underwater course using the same rebreather equipment, unbeknown to him other divers began resurfacing with the same symptoms. Oblivious, Sparky stubbornly continued trying to complete as many circuits as he could in the inky blackness of the freezing water, despite once more being overcome with agonising headaches and chest pains.

'I caught up with another diver, stopped on the wire,' Sparky told me. 'I thought he was just struggling or knackered and having a rest. I found out later he was having the same problems as me and was just trying to sort his breathing out. I pushed on past him totally unaware. I thought I was the only one having these problems.'

Ultimately a thunder flash – a large industrial firework – was thrown into the water by the instructors, the sonic shockwave when it exploded was the unmistakable emergency signal to bring all the divers immediately to the surface. With one diver after another resurfacing and complaining of the same problems, the instructors had realised something was desperately wrong and belatedly ended the exercise.

Sparky resurfaced to see ambulances already in place on the shore waiting for them. Almost everyone had been affected. Having been the first person to resurface with problems he'd then, crucially, been sent back down again. None of the other divers who surfaced with problems were sent back. He'd been down twice, much longer than anyone else and exposed to whatever was wrong for far longer. The devastating effects of that prolonged exposure would prove life-changing for Sparky.

CHAPTER 16

ABANDONED

After the diving incident and a brief stay in hospital for tests and to recover, Sparky and his colleagues were discharged. They were never told what the problem had been. In the weeks and months that followed, Sparky noticed the first problems with his eyesight.

Despite the diving episode, having gone on to pass the selection course Sparky was accepted onto the next SC3 course, and shortly after began training proper to become a member of the SBS.

'There was a lot of bookwork, stuff to learn about diving,' he explained over another pint. 'I was still trying to study late at night when everybody else had finished. Even then I was using a magnifying glass to help with my reading. It was a bloody night-mare. I couldn't keep up. Nobody could understand why I was struggling. Including me.'

Eventually, he took himself to a private optician to see if they could help. After a basic eye test, he was told he had a 'lazy eye'. He was advised to wear an eye patch over the good eye to build the strength up in the lazy one.

'Well, as you can imagine, Mick, that really wasn't an option on an SC's course. If I'd turned to in the morning looking like a pirate, they'd have laughed me out of camp.'

Sparky reluctantly decided to remove himself from the course, planning to sort the problem out and, once fully fit, complete the course in the future.

'I got a lot of grief,' he said. 'I couldn't really give them a good reason why I was dropping out. I obviously couldn't tell the officer in charge the real reason – the last thing I wanted was to be medically downgraded. I just said I didn't feel ready for it yet. The OC was really disappointed and couldn't work out why I wanted to leave as I was doing well. On my personal docs it says, "withdrew himself from SC3s training for no apparent reason". I thought I'd go away, sort the lazy eye problem out, then everything would be OK. Sadly, it didn't work out that way.'

His eye condition steadily worsened. Acutely aware of this and desperate to save his career, Sparky decided to volunteer for a signals course. He thought this would be a branch where he could still maintain his soldiering while at the same time be able to compensate for his deteriorating vision.

'All the time I still thought it was going to get better, but I was terrified they'd medically downgrade me if they found out. That meant becoming a clerk or a chef in those days. That would have killed me. I thought the sigs branch would give me somewhere to continue my career while my sight recovered. I'd find somewhere to hide while things improved. All I wanted was to stay in the corps. It was my life. It didn't quite work out like that, though.'

Despite his steadily worsening vision, Sparky managed to get through his signals course, as always, and despite his increasing disability, excelling. Until the final exercise.

By that time he needed a magnifying glass to read pretty much anything. 'On the final exercise, which was in the field and tactical, the only way I could read and fill in the radio log at night was to use a tiny pen torch and my magnifying glass. Long story short, I got bumped by the instructor. A naked light in a tactical position: unthinkable. I'd compromised the whole fucking exercise,' he explained. 'Instant failure.'

'I got the bollocking of my life afterwards. The chief instructor screaming at me, wanting to know why a bloke with my experience would behave in such an unprofessional manner. Telling me I should be ashamed. In the end I just gave up. I told him, "I can't see, sir. There's something wrong with my eyes." '

'You can't see?' the officer questioned in disbelief. 'What do you mean you can't see?'

Sparky explained that his eyesight had been deteriorating for well over a year, that he wasn't able to read without a magnifying glass, that he could only see shapes. It was the first time he'd admitted the truth to anyone and it felt like a weight lifted from his shoulders. It wasn't. The officer in charge didn't believe him. He thought it was a feeble excuse to cover his actions on the final exercise.

'Get down to the sick bay and get an eye test now,' he ordered.

At the sick bay things went from bad to worse. He was put in front of an eye chart by the Royal Naval medical assistant on duty and asked to read the letters. He could make little out beneath the top two lines. When he explained this, the MA refused to believe him.

'You do know faking a disability is a chargeable offence, don't you?'

'I'm not faking anything. I can't read anything below the top two lines.'

The MA moved Sparky closer to the chart. 'How about now?'

'The same. I can't make out anything but shapes below the top two lines.'

'If you're trying to work your ticket,' the MA said slowly, thinking Sparky was after a medical discharge, 'it's not going to happen. I can tell you that now.'

'Work my ticket?' Sparky shouted. 'I can't fucking see! What do you want me to say?'

Amazingly, still nobody believed him. Even worse, they didn't know what to do with him. He was removed from the signals course and given a series of jobs around the camp, to keep him occupied while they worked out what the solution was.

'Believe it or not, Mick' – he stopped and laughed – 'they ended up making me the safety look out at Straight Point Ranges. Can you imagine, a blind man responsible to check if ships are sailing across a rifle range? I couldn't even make out the dots on the radar let alone see if any boats were at sea fouling the range. You couldn't make it up, could you?'

As farcical as it was, that job finally brought a turning point to Sparky's worsening situation. Unable to judge accurately if the range was fouled or not and conscious someone could be killed if he allowed firing to take place when a ship or fishing boat strayed onto the range, Sparky simply raised the red Range Fouled flag if there was the slightest doubt in his mind, which was often. That meant firing was constantly being halted on the range with a resulting backlog of troops unable to complete their weapons tests.

'The weapons instructors hated me, Mick' – Sparky grimaced – 'but what could I do? I didn't want someone to get shot because I couldn't see bugger all.'

Eventually, because of the increasing delays on the range and the resulting complaints, Sparky was hauled before a medical review board. They were looking to take disciplinary action against him for malingering. Amazingly, still nobody believed he had a problem with his sight.

Then fate took a hand.

'They marched me in and stood me to attention in front of the review board, which was at a desk at one end of the room. I thought I was going to be locked up, kicked out or both. But who do you think was the officer presiding over the review board?' he asked.

'No idea, mate,' I replied.

'Dr Rick Jolly, from the Falklands.' He grinned.

Rick Jolly spent some time looking carefully through Sparky's file before looking up. 'I know you, Marine Sparkes, don't I?'

'We've met sir,' Sparky replied, and reminded him of when he handed his injured patrol member over to him in the Falklands.

'Yes, I remember,' the doctor replied.

He looked through the files in front of him.

'But this makes no sense. I'm being told there's nothing wrong with you, that you're malingering. But with your history, that's nonsense.'

He continued to flick through the files then turned to the three Royal Navy officers, side by side, who were stood at ease to the right of Sparky. They were the medical officers who'd been responsible for his care, who claimed there was nothing wrong with him.

'I can't find Marine Sparkes ophthalmic examination results. Are they in here?' he queried.

The senior of the three officers took the file and searched through it. Fruitlessly. 'I can't seem to find it,' he said, 'but it must be in here somewhere.'

'I'm presuming he has had an ophthalmic examination?' Rick Jolly questioned suspiciously.

'Of course, he must have. It will be in here somewhere, sir,' the increasingly flustered officer replied.

Finally out of patience, Rick Jolly said, 'I'll settle this problem for you. Marine Sparkes. Have you ever had an ophthalmic examination?'

There was a pause before Sparky answered. 'No, sir. No, sir, I haven't.'

It had been almost a year since Sparky had admitted to the problems he was having with his vision and in all that time the medical department had never once given him a full ophthalmic examination.

Rick Jolly went ballistic. 'You three have treated this man like a piece of meat! Get out of my sight! Now! I'll deal with you later!'

Rick Jolly promptly rang Haslar, the Royal Navy hospital in Gosport near Portsmouth. The facility, appropriately enough, was named after Major 'Blondie' Haslar, commanding officer of the Cockleshell Heroes. Within a few hours Sparky found himself transported to the hospital and undergoing his first ever full ophthalmic examination. It was progress at long last. It was more than two-and-a-half years since the diving incident which seemed to trigger Sparky's visual impairment and a year since he'd admitted he was losing his sight. For the first time, finally somebody believed him.

'I can't tell you exactly what you're suffering from, Marine Sparkes,' said the doctor who carried out the test at Haslar later that day. 'But I'm afraid to say I can tell you there is something very seriously wrong with your eyes.'

The joy of his condition being at long last acknowledged was at once replaced with the gut-wrenching realisation of its severity.

CHAPTER 17

THE LIGHT AT THE END OF A VERY LONG TUNNEL

With his deteriorating eyesight finally acknowledged, Sparky could have been excused for thinking his problems might finally be coming to an end. That couldn't have been further from the truth. With little in place in the mid-1980s to support him within the military, Sparky found himself with an uncertain future ahead.

'They basically sent me on extended leave while they tried to work out what they were going to do with me. I was just trying to stay fit and positive and hopefully find a way to stay in the corps, but my eyes were getting worse.'

He told me a story that was typical of his relentlessly positive approach, and how he coped with that uncertain time. To keep fit he used to regularly run around the lanes surrounding Commando Training Centre Royal Marines (CTCRM) near where he lived when on this extended leave.

The lanes around the camp are narrow, lined with banks, often single tracked with passing points. Because troops are regularly running and marching along them, locals drive cautiously. Sparky could still make out the shape of the banks with his peripheral vision and he knew the area, so he felt confident running around the roads.

One day, on one of these regular training runs, he heard a car engine ahead. He knew he was approaching a passing point, so he speeded up to reach it before the oncoming vehicle.

'I thought I'd just sprint into the little layby I knew was ahead, stop and let the car go by. What I didn't know was there was a woman riding a horse in front of me who'd had the same idea and she was already there. I was running along fine then all of a sudden something big and warm hit me in the face. My legs flew forwards. I fell flat on my back, totally winded. I'd run straight up the horse's arse and was now sprawled out beneath it. All I could hear was the horse whinnying like crazy as it reared up. The rider trying desperately to stay in the saddle, calling me all the names under the sun. Then the next thing I know, the car we'd both been trying to avoid drives up and stops next to me there on the ground. The bloke inside winds down his window, leans out and shouts, "That is the funniest thing I have ever seen in my life," then drives off laughing his head off.'

Although his Royal Marine career seemed doomed, his sight problems at least were finally being investigated. There was a problem, though. Sparky had been so effective in covering his increasingly worsening eyesight that it was two-and-a-half years after the diving incident and Sparky's first symptoms before anyone began actively investigating. To cloud the waters more, there was also no record of Sparky or anybody else being taken to hospital directly after the equipment problem. There had even been a court of enquiry directly after the incident, where Sparky and the other divers affected had been called as witnesses. However, they were never told the result or any findings, and once more there were no records available.

'They weren't prepared to accept that the diving episode was the cause, so they decided I had a genetic fault and that I had Stargardt disease,' Sparky told me.

Stargardt is a rare form of macular degeneration which affects the retinas in both eyes. It causes a loss of vision in the central part of the eye, the part that deals with detail and colour, facial recognition and reading. Although macular degeneration in general is more common in the elderly, Stargardt primarily affects juveniles, adolescents and young adults.

If there was a positive side to the diagnosis it was that although his macular vision was steadily deteriorating, his peripheral vision was unaffected and would probably remain so. He could still make out blurry outlines and shapes. Most likely he would not lose his sight completely. It was an oasis of good news in a desert of bad.

That must have been how he'd been able to hide the problem so effectively for so long. His limited peripheral vision meant he'd been able to find a way to function. It may have also explained why people, at least initially, had found it difficult to believe he was telling the truth when he finally admitted to his failing eyesight.

The fact that he'd fought so hard and so long to cope meant that any connection with the long-ago diving incident could be disputed. The timeframe and the lack of medical records allowed the system deniability in terms of any liability. This was the cheapest solution for the system, but not necessarily the best solution for Sparky.

Some months later Sparky was ordered to return from extended leave to attend a review board in Plymouth. Given no prior indication as to the reason for the review, he was marched in and unceremoniously informed that his career was over. He was medically discharged that day.

To make matters worse, despite having qualified for promotion to full corporal and the date for him to be promoted having already passed, Sparky was discharged at the lower rank of marine, which meant a much lower pension.

'Career over, no job, home, no money and going blind,' Sparky told me angrily. 'I went back to camp, threw my green beret on my bed and cried my eyes out.'

No rehabilitation training was offered. No connection with organisations to help blind veterans proffered. Nothing was done to help ease him into the life that lay ahead of him coping with his disability. Sparky was on his own.

When Sparky told me his incredible story, all within the first couple of hours of meeting him again in The Coach House, I was speechless. Although I'd known about his sight loss, I hadn't been aware of any of the details surrounding it. I'd most certainly never heard how poorly he'd been treated.

'What did you do then?' I asked.

'Ten years later I ended up married with a beautiful daughter – Stephania – living in Malta. I was selling timeshares. Before they got a bad name!' He laughed. 'I was good at it. My macular vision had totally gone by then though and it's quite hard to sell timeshares when you can't see. Makes filling the forms in a lot harder. I was struggling to get by. To be honest, I was almost at the end of my tether. Then a lady called Mrs Bloomer contacted me, and for the first time in a long time things started to look up.'

Mrs Bloomer was connected to SSAFA – the Soldiers, Sailors Airforce Families Association – the oldest tri-service charity in the UK. She was English but lived on Malta, and she'd heard of Sparky through the close-knit Maltese community. She met him and told him she wanted to help him get support for his disability. It was a decade after his discharge from the Royal Marines and the first time anyone had specifically offered to help him deal with his sight loss. She put him in touch with Blind Veterans UK, known then as St Dunstan's. They were and remain, under their new name, the principle charity in Britain dealing with veteran's sight loss.

'They flew me back to the UK for a week's rehabilitation training at their centre just up the road,' Sparky said, gesturing. 'It was like someone had turned the lights back on again for me. After that I decided to relocate back to the UK permanently and complete the full rehabilitation programme with them. I lived at the centre for the next eighteen months, learning to live and work with my sight loss. They saved my life, Mick, no question about it – Mrs Bloomer and Blind Veterans saved my life.'

The first thing Blind Veterans did when they repatriated Sparky was to try to address his pension situation. They sent him to another ophthalmic doctor to confirm what the issues were and if they could relate to the diving incident. He confirmed there were cases in the US Navy Seal teams of individuals suffering similar effects in similar situations to the ones experienced by Sparky. It was basically oxygen starvation.

'It may or may not have caused the problem,' Sparky told me, 'but at the very least it would have aggravated it, the doctor said.'

It seemed at long last that Sparky was finally about to receive the support and the compensation which he was entitled too.

The charity approached the Ministry of Defence on Sparky's behalf with the new medical findings, full of confidence. They were swiftly informed that the 1997 Army Act had recently come into force. Now, no one could revisit a pre-existing medical condition more than three years after their final service date. Over a decade after his discharge, Sparky was well outside that criteria. Frustratingly, though, he'd missed his window to put things right over ten years later by little more than a whisker, as it was just weeks after the Army Act had come into force. It didn't matter how strong his argument was now or what proof he had, he had no legal right to take the MOD to court to challenge their findings. His case was closed.

I couldn't believe what had happened to Sparky, but most of all I couldn't believe how the system had so completely abandoned him. A lesser man would have been dead by now.

Darren, The Coach House landlord, came over for a chat.

'Has any blind person rowed an ocean, Mick?' he asked out of the blue, well aware of my ocean rowing background.

It took me by surprise. I thought for a minute and then answered, 'I don't think so, mate. Not that I'm aware of.' (I'd find out later when I looked into it that a blind veteran who was in fact a friend of Sparky's had already rowed the Atlantic Ocean.)

'Why don't you and Sparky row one, then?' he said casually, as if suggesting a Sunday walk on the nearby Sussex Downs.

Sparky laughed. I smiled. Inside, though, the moment it was mentioned it felt as if a light switch had been flicked. A blind man rowing an ocean would be an incredible story. He could become an inspiration for a huge number of people struggling with all manner of problems, not just sight loss.

I'd never imagined wanting to row another ocean after the North Pacific crossing to the Golden Gate Bridge in 2009. I didn't think I could ever surpass that achievement. But I knew the moment it was suggested I should row with Sparky that that had changed – I knew I should go rowing again. It was as instant and as certain as that.

Once more, it seemed, luck had brought me back onto the path I was meant to be on.

'I'm up for it if you are, mate,' I finally said.

Sparky carried on laughing for a few seconds. Then asked, 'Are you serious?'

'Yeah, why not? You're more than capable of doing it. I'm out of work now anyhow, so I need a project. It'll be a laugh, you'll love it.'

He thought for a while then the trace of a grin spread across his face. 'If you can make it happen, mate, I'm in.'

'Leave it with me,' I said, much more confident than I actually was, 'I'll get it sorted.'

I had no clue exactly how I was going to do that.

*　　*　　*

The next day Sparky woke up to the joys of a well-earned hangover before, later in the day, receiving the news that I'd found a boat and we were going to row across the Pacific from California to Hawaii, almost three thousand miles, in the Great Pacific Race.

'It will be a great project and you'll be an inspiration,' I told him. 'Most importantly, mate, it's an opportunity to replace a little of what losing your sight has robbed you of. You'll be the first blind person to row the Pacific. There's only ever one first. That should be you.'

'So, when is it?'

'Next June. We've got nine months.'

'Bloody hell! I suppose I'd better start learning to row.'

CHAPTER 18

NOTHING LIKE A TIGHT DEADLINE!

Having committed to rowing across the Pacific with Sparky, there was now the small matter of making it happen. We had little more than eight months to put everything in place. We needed to get a boat, kit it out and have it ready for shipping to the US by March 2018. Sparky needed training to be ready to row an ocean and there was substantial expenditure to find a budget for. This included the race entry fee, boat shipping (to the US and back from Hawaii), boat costs, kit costs, flights, accommodation and a hundred other expenses that come with such a major undertaking.

As confident as I always tried to appear on the outside, I thought I might have finally bitten off more than I could chew. I never considered I'd made a mistake – I was doing the right thing, I was certain. I simply wasn't sure exactly how I was going to make it work this time. In the past I'd always had a certain amount of disposable finance of my own to make up for any shortfall in the project budget. Now I had none. The project had to stand completely on its own feet, and within such a tight timeframe I wasn't convinced that was possible.

Ideally there would have been a two-year build up to a project as ambitious as this. We didn't have that luxury. If we missed the deadline for the next Great Pacific Race in June 2018, it was a further two years before the race was due to be run again. The moment would pass; it would be too easy for it never to happen. I knew it was now or never.

*   *   *

The morning after our evening in the pub, I'd spoken to the organisers of the Atlantic rowing race to see if that might be an alternative option for us. They informed me that we could enter, but only in a four-man team. They pointed out that, Sparky being blind, he wouldn't be able to keep a look out. I asked them who kept watch on their solo boats in the Atlantic race when the rower slept? Surely the technology they would rely on to keep them safe from collision while they slept would protect Sparky while he was on deck? They didn't have an answer for that, but regardless they remained unmoved. They'd be happy to have us take part but only in a four.

A four defeated the object. We were trying to demonstrate that being blind doesn't have to limit your capability to realise your ambitions and achieve your goals. If Sparky was put on a boat effectively as a passenger, all we would be demonstrating was that he was very much limited by his disability.

As luck would have it, I then discovered that Sparky's friend from Blind Veterans, Alan Lock, former Royal Navy, had already rowed the Atlantic, so it became a moot point. But I was disappointed at the organisers' attitude. Ocean rowing had always been about a diverse group of people achieving seemingly impossible goals. It seemed to me that their decision flew in the face of that tradition.

So I rang my old friend Chris Martin, who I'd rowed the North Pacific with in 2009. He was the director of the Great Pacific Race – from Monterey Bay, 2400 nautical miles (the shortest possible distance, seldom achieved) to Honolulu. It wasn't quite the seven-thousand-mile epic voyage we'd completed together from Japan to San Francisco, but it was still a formidable challenge, and no blind person had yet rowed the Pacific.

'It would be better if you went in a four, Mick,' was Chris's initial response.

'Yeah, oddly enough that's already been mentioned, mate,' I replied dryly. 'That's not an option, as this is about showing what a blind person is capable of. That won't work if he's just a passenger on a four. He's perfectly capable of rowing in a double and being successful.'

'Right' – Chris paused, thinking for a few seconds – 'a pair it is then. It would have put my mind at ease if it was a four, but I get your point and as its you . . .' – he laughed. 'Welcome to the Great Pacific Race, mate. Great to have you and Sparky on board.'

I had a race, now I needed a boat. Chris mentioned a couple of suitable boats that were available for rent and which would come almost ready to go. The costs were prohibitive, though. There was only one boat I really wanted to return to the Pacific with and that was *Bo*, the fabulous rowing boat I had built specifically to cross the North Pacific in 2009.

I contacted Daryl Farmer, who I'd sold *Bo* to a few years earlier, and asked if he had any plans for her or if she might be available to buy or rent for the race.

Daryl had only recently returned from a successful solo crossing of the Atlantic with *Bo*. 'I've never thought of renting her before, to be honest. Not sure I'd trust anyone with her. You're a different matter, though – I know you'll look after her,' he said, chuckling. 'I'm more than happy to work out a way for you to have her back for the race, Mick. It would be another great chapter in her story and I'd be glad to help make it happen.'

So, with a race entry in place and a boat, all I needed now was a budget to pay for it all. At a conservative estimate, I knew it was going to run well into the tens of thousands of pounds. What I didn't know though was how I was going to find that kind of money in such an incredibly short space of time.

I was lucky: as with the race entry and *Bo*'s return, there were a lot of people who wanted to help. Many of them, fortunately, drank in The Coach House in Rottingdean, the birthplace of the whole project. Much as my family pub, The Cowbridge, in my hometown of Boston had become the HQ for my earlier ocean rowing projects, The Coach took on that role for my and Sparky's Pacific adventure.

Darren and Hayley, the landlord and landlady, immediately got behind the project. From charity fundraisers to connecting with local sponsors, they could not have done more to give the project a fighting chance of success. As it was Darren's innocent, if loaded, question about a blind person having rowed an ocean which started the whole thing, it could be argued it was perhaps the least they could do. Nonetheless, it was a massive help and kept the momentum going, which the project seemed to gather immediately from its inception, growing steadily.

A group of regulars from The Coach, local businessmen with whom I'd become good friends over the years, immediately offered their support. The principle gang of three who threw their weight behind the project were Big Frank, an ex-BBC camera man who now runs his own media film company, FC Media; Dave Bull, a senior manager in the Ambulance Service and ex-Army; and Dave Sutton, a former fisherman who had his own boat building company. They'd had the misfortune to be in the pub the night I met Sparky again. Like Sparky, they thought it sounded like a great idea at the time and happily offered their support as the beer flowed. Also, like Sparky, they woke the next day, somewhat worse for wear, surprised to discover the vaguely remembered scheme from the previous night wasn't just beer talk and plans were already well under way for its execution.

I'm happy to say it didn't dampen their enthusiasm for the project, nor change their mind about supporting it. As a result of their early financial backing, we had at least enough in the kitty to get us up and running, and we also had practical support in the shape of refitting *Bo* at Dave Sutton's boatyard. As the project progressed, it would be no exaggeration to say that, without their support, and Big Frank's support in particular, the project would have folded long before the start line. There would be a long, hard and steep road ahead of us simply to reach California, let alone Hawaii, but these guys were there from day one to make sure we made it.

I realised Sparky becoming the first visually impaired person to row the Pacific could potentially generate a massive amount of positive publicity. It could be a golden opportunity for any charity to benefit from a partnership both in terms of raising awareness and raising funds for their own aims. More importantly, from a selfish point of view, a charity could potentially bring the contacts and exposure we would need to help fund our formidable budget.

Fortunately, thanks to Keith Breslauer's introduction, I'd already worked consistently with The Royal Marines Charity during my kayaking expeditions with Steve Grenham. We'd built up a great relationship. They'd supported all of the kayaking adventures and, through those adventures, we'd managed to raise enough money to purchase and donate a number of folding kayaks to the Royal Marines Kayaking Association for recovering veterans to use in future expeditions and races.

The Royal Marines Charity are a proactive and efficient modern charity. They are doing their very best to provide a vital service to those members of the Royal Marines family, serving and former, and their dependants, who need their help. It's an organisation that hadn't existed in Sparky's time, or I'm sure his story would have been very different. I was more than happy to continue that partnership so long, of course, as they wished to be connected with our Pacific plans.

Sparky owed his life to Blind Veterans UK. Since catching up with Sparky again, I went to see the incredible work they do on a daily basis at their local centre in Ovingdean. Since they were such a central part of Sparky's story, I thought they really should be involved in his latest and biggest adventure.

We arranged a meeting between both charities, me and Sparky to discuss the possibilities at the start of October. Everyone was enthusiastic about the project but, equally, everyone was anxious about the short timeframe. Including me. I knew exactly what was required and I knew that time was now our most precious commodity. I emphasised how quickly the New Year would come and the months we currently had to prepare would soon become weeks. We had to work fast to make it happen. It was doable, but we needed proactive and enthusiastic partners to help get us to the start line. The work needed to start now.

In many ways, the most important partners would be the two charities. We could deliver the row; I had no doubt about that. We'd get the boat to Hawaii, but we'd need both charities, with their infrastructure and expertise, to maximise publicity and fundraising for the charities, to make it something of even greater value than just two blokes rowing to Hawaii, even if one of the blokes happened to be blind. We couldn't generate that extra value on our own.

The Royal Marines Charity representative couldn't have been more positive. As soon as I'd outlined what was in place, our capabilities, what was required and the potential the project had, he said, 'We're in if Blind Vets are.' The representative for Blind Veterans UK, although equally as enthusiastic about the project, was not quite so convinced.

At no point did I or Sparky ever doubt that we'd be physically and mentally capable of completing what we were striving to achieve, despite Sparky's disability. We were former Royal Marines, both still fit, and I had a huge amount of experience on ocean rowing boats. We would simply compensate for Sparky's lack of sight as a team. As the meeting progressed, the Blind Veterans representative suddenly turned to Sparky and said, 'But Sparky, do you really think you're up to this? This is going to be incredibly tough. Two months or more on a rowing boat with your condition?'

Sparky barely reacted. He'd obviously spent decades proving people wrong and silencing the doubters, so it was water off a duck's back to him. I, on the other hand, quickly became offended on his behalf.

'Sparky's only lost his sight,' I said indignant. 'He has a hundred qualities anyone else in the race can only dream of. Sparky wasn't just a Royal Marine; he was an exceptional Royal Marine. Those qualities don't disappear. He'll have no problem successfully completing this. Trust me.'

Eventually we did get the support of both charities, and the momentum continued to build. The clock was ticking but we were on track and on target. We couldn't ask for more than that.

CHAPTER 19

HEARTBREAK

By the time I agreed to row the Pacific with Sparky, my wife, Grace, and I had been together for over ten years. We'd met and married in Nigeria when I'd worked there for three years, preparing for my North Pacific row in 2009. Although we were very happy together, I'm under no illusion I was the easiest of men to be married to. Within two weeks of our wedding I'd set off on the North Pacific row with Chris. Grace and I then didn't see each other again for almost another nine months. Unhelpful and inflexible immigration laws both in the UK and Nigeria conspired to keep us apart even longer after my return from the Pacific. She had to endure an awful lot to be with me.

After we eventually set up home in the UK, I'm sure she hoped the ocean rowing adventures were behind me. I thought they were – I had never imagined rowing an ocean again. I didn't think anything could eclipse what Chris and I achieved on the North Pacific.

Grace was unhappy and disappointed when I embarked on the Cockleshell Endeavour paddling exploits with Steve, but eventually came to recognise the good they were doing. In fact, she was the person who noticed the difference most in Steve. She'd found him distant and unapproachable when she first met him. Even intimidating. By the end of the project, she looked on him like a brother. 'He's like a different person,' she'd said. Despite that, when I told her about Sparky and the plans to cross the Pacific, her reaction was very different.

Grace was by that stage in full-time education studying for a degree. She made it clear she didn't want the added financial pressure another ocean rowing project would bring.

I understood her concerns but, equally, I'd been reluctant to disappear abroad again to work, rarely getting home. I'd finished my contract on the yacht in the US early in 2017. That job saw me return home fewer than six weeks in thirteen months. I'd planned to return to sailing with the job in St Bart's, but, in truth, part of the appeal of rowing with Sparky was the possibility of creating another way forwards, one which might allow me, eventually, to have something approaching a normal home life. At least, normal by my standards.

I'd already begun to expand on my motivational and keynote speaking work, which I based around my ocean rowing adventures and the innumerable lessons learned and how they translated into the business world. I was gaining a good reputation and beginning to generate a modest income from it. It didn't compare to a captain's salary on a private yacht, but potentially, as it grew, it had the scope to dwarf it. I'd just published my first book, *Rowing the Pacific*, which was receiving excellent reviews and was on sale worldwide. I already had a Discovery Channel documentary covering the 2009 row to my name, and I was creating an impressive CV, which I was confident I could build on. A successful row across the Pacific with Sparky, I thought, would allow me to write another book and possibly produce a second documentary.

Most importantly, as well as a new career path away from professional sailing, I wanted to build on the Cockleshell Endeavour concept. I was passionate about creating a permanent resource for recovering veterans under that banner. The goal was to use the same simple principles we'd used working with Steve Grenham to get veterans who were having issues, either physical or mental, back on track. Likeminded people, with a shared history, completing water or ocean-based projects, races and expeditions together. Getting people to communicate, getting them fit, engaged and energised again.

It was a simple concept, but we'd seen how well it worked. If I could recreate this on a larger, sustainable scale, it could have impressive results and produce something of real value and meaning. I was confident I could succeed. The Pacific row with Sparky could be the perfect launch pad for all of these plans, as well as being an incredible project in its own right. Losing the job in St Bart's, thanks to Hurricane Irma's destructive legacy, was, I believed, yet another fateful intervention, one which which had sent me back on the path I was meant to be on.

Grace was much more of a realist. Growing up in Nigeria, she'd had an incredibly tough life compared to mine. She rightly craved security and a future that was risk free. It seemed to me that she didn't understand what I was trying to achieve, and she didn't believe in it. It was heart-breaking when this became obvious.

Life had been particularly tough for us as a couple for a few years leading up to this. With hindsight, I'd certainly been guilty of not fully recognising how tough it had been for Grace. Sometimes a positive attitude and just getting on with life is not the best way forwards. I should have been a more understanding husband. I'd always been a difficult person to be married to, but it was now becoming apparent that Grace had grown to feel I was thoughtless and selfish. She probably had a good point. Problems which had obviously been fermenting just below the surface of our relationship for some time now came to the fore. Our mutual desires to pursue very different ambitions and career paths, and ultimately different lives, sadly signalled the end of our relationship. Grace handed me divorce papers and made it clear our marriage was over.

It was a devastating turn of events, one for which I hold myself totally responsible. Grace is a unique and wonderful person who

I loved dearly. I'd never considered we wouldn't grow old together. I realised, though, that I wasn't providing the life for her she longed for and I never would. I wasn't the person she needed to share her life with. In fact, I was probably the complete opposite.

I was always going to want to row oceans and look for more adventures. Nine-to-five would be the definition of a death sentence for me. I had absolute belief in what I was trying to achieve and I knew I was meant to pursue that path. I'd lived the whole of my adult life listening to those instincts. If I turned my back on them now, they would only return to haunt me further down the road.

CHAPTER 20

GOOD THINGS COME IN THREES

Despite great support for the Cockleshell Pacific Endeavour, I still needed to find substantial funding to cover the major bills on the horizon, and I found myself crushed beneath the combined weight of the project and the collapse of my marriage. I thought I might finally have bitten off more than I could chew with my latest rowing adventure. As September drifted into October, it felt like I was suffocating under the pressure.

Fatefully, three unconnected but very important events conspired to drag me back from the brink of abject despair. Steve Grenham provided the first.

Blind Veterans UK invited me and Sparky to attend a boxing dinner being held at a Brighton Hotel. A local boxing club was fighting the Royal Marines boxing squad. It was a fundraiser for both of our charities and a chance to promote the row. I invited Steve Grenham along; it was his first opportunity to meet Sparky. It was a successful night, and a lot of fun. Afterwards, Steve Grenham and I stopped for a drink in a nearby pub.

Steve asked out of the blue, 'So? How are you doing, then?'

I didn't really know how to answer that. At the time I didn't think I'd ever been 'doing' worse.

I tried to waffle a response, saying everything was getting sorted, it was a bad time, but things would work out. He saw straight through it.

'I asked how you were doing? Don't give me all that shit.'

I smiled. It was actually a relief that someone thought I might be having a tough time and wanted to know about it. I had relentlessly tried to maintain an outwardly positive approach. My situation was of my own making, a result of my own choices; there was no point moaning about things that were my responsibility and certainly no point telling anyone about them. Now, it suddenly became very appealing to unload some of the pressure.

'Honestly, mate? I'm fucked. My marriage is over, and I live in a room behind my mate's office. Work's not great and I've got a rowing project to deliver with no money to make it happen . . . All in all, it's not been my best year.'

It felt like a weight lifted just saying it out loud.

Steve, always straight to the point, nodded and replied matter-of-factly, 'Don't worry about all the shitty stuff – that will sort itself out in time. Make this Pacific thing happen. You made all our Cockleshell Endeavour stuff happen and that changed my life. I can already see this doing the same for Sparky. Stop worrying about it and just make it happen. Everything else will fall into place, mate.'

I was taken aback, embarrassed, humbled and flattered all at the same time. It wasn't the response I'd expected. I knew our paddling exploits had been a success and had made a positive impact on Steve, but to hear him say it changed his life? It left me speechless and, if I'm honest, a little choked. For him to add that making the Pacific project happen was the right decision and what I should be doing had a profound impact – I needed to hear that. Belief flooded back into me. I hadn't fully realised it, but I'd been on a spiral towards disaster and failure. Steve Grenham and that one conversation halted that spiral down.

An unexpected conversation with Natalie Harper just a few weeks later would have just as powerful an impact. It wouldn't just help to halt that spiral down – it would put me on an upward trajectory towards success.

I'd known Natalie Harper for several years but only to say hi to in The Coach. She was best friends with Hayley, the landlady. My first real conversation with her came when she mentioned she was going to climb Mount Kilimanjaro.

'I didn't realise you were a climber,' I said.

'I'm not,' she replied, laughing. 'About a dozen of us came up with the idea a year ago. Since then everybody but me and one friend has dropped out. I said I'd do it, though, so I'm going to do it.'

Listening to her made me smile. It sounded exactly like something I'd say.

I offered to lend her some kit for the trip, including a satellite tracker so her family could follow her progress throughout the climb. I knew from experience how important that would be for the people back home and how much extra interest it could generate for her project.

When she finally disappeared to Tanzania to complete her adventure, following Nat's exploits climbing Kilimanjaro became a welcome distraction for me. The tracker proved a great success, as family and friends back home religiously followed her daily progress up the mountain. Eight days after she set off, on 18 October, Nat summited the highest free-standing mountain in the world – Mount Kilimanjaro, the roof of Africa. She returned rightly proud of her accomplishment. The fact that she'd completed it simply because she had said she would made her success even more impressive in my eyes.

After her descent she sent me a photograph. It was Nat and her friend standing proudly at the summit of the mountain, Nat holding a copy of *Rowing the Pacific* in her hand. In the message she thanked me for the loan of the tracker and told me she loved the book. 'It got me through the tough times reading it,' she wrote. Her message and the picture were a welcome ray of sunshine in what was increasingly becoming a very dark time for me.

On her return, Nat was keen to repay the favour and help with the preparation for the Pacific. I was glad of the offer. Her infectious enthusiasm and drive were a welcome addition, as I was still labouring under the 'mountain' I had to climb: getting Sparky and me to the start of the Great Pacific Race. As much as the spiral down had halted after Steve Grenham's words, the practical realities hadn't changed. I was still looking at huge bills to pay in the very near future with no real budget in place to cover them. I confided in Nat just how tough it was becoming and the doubts which were once again beginning to creep in.

'You have to do this, Mick,' she said. 'Look how much you've done already. You've got a boat, you're in the race, the charities are behind you, sponsorship's growing. The rest will fall into place. This is what you do, Mick. I know you'll make this happen. And anyhow, I'm already planning on coming to Hawaii to see you finish.'

Much like the unexpected conversation with Steve Grenham, I was once again taken by surprise but for different reasons. I couldn't understand how someone who didn't really know me that well could have such faith in me.

'Ahh!' she said, laughing. 'You forget, Mick. I've read your book.' Looking back now, I realise that was the first indication we were becoming more than just friends.

It was another crucial turning point for me, just when I needed it most. Two simple conversations only a few weeks apart changed my perception of the situation completely. It's essential to have belief in yourself, but when things become tough, really tough, other people's belief in you has a value way beyond that. It's what keeps you going when you think you're done.

*   *   *

With my confidence and belief gratefully restored, I set about repaying Steve and Nat's faith in me with renewed vigour. I'd make it happen. I still wasn't sure how, but I'd find a way.

As luck would have it, the way found me. Not long after those conversations with Steve and Nat I received an unexpected phone call from an old mate, Luke Francis. Luke was another former marine who I'd worked with for a time providing armed escorts on ships transiting Somalia when the piracy problem in the Indian Ocean was at its height. He was a different generation of marine to me, younger and a product of the Afghan conflict, but a great bloke. We'd become good friends.

'I hear you've got another project, mate,' he said.

'Yep, I'm going to row the Pacific with a blind bootneck,' I replied.

'How's sponsorship going?'

'Not good.'

'I think I might have some good news for you, then,' he said.

He wasn't exaggerating. He introduced me to his old friend Paul Moynan, another former marine. Paul had left the corps and had cofounded Dragon Coin, one of the leading lights in the new blockchain technology boom. He was actively looking to support projects to promote the Dragon Coin ethos. He loved what we were doing and wanted to sponsor us. In fact, he wanted to be the title sponsor. It was a very welcome early Christmas present.

Once again, I was speechless as the reality sank in. It was almost too good to be true. I had gone from despair, not knowing where the next penny was coming from to get us to the start line, to putting in place a large chunk of the total budget of the project. It remained to be seen if we'd make it to Hawaii, but we were most certainly going to California. Good things did, it seem, come in threes, and apparently when you least expect them.

CHAPTER 21

AMERICA

With Dragon Coin's very welcome title sponsorship falling into place just before the New Year, it meant we could now reliably plan for the trip to America. I still needed to find more funding, but we'd broken the back of the budget issues. I arrived in America a few days earlier than Sparky to drum up support for the project in San Francisco. I gave a couple of presentations at yacht clubs and local organisations, and set up some book signings to help promote our plans. I had a lot of friends in the city who were all keen to support us. I picked Sparky up the day he flew into San Francisco and we drove down the coast to the start in Monterey.

Bo had arrived in Monterey a couple of days earlier – we'd arranged for the race organiser to collect her from the container port and tow her to the start on her trailer. There was still a lot of work to do to have her ready for sea, so it was going to be a frantic build up to the race. She'd been stripped down and packed for a journey in a shipping container, and now we had to restore her to being a fully functioning ocean rowing boat.

As much as Dragon's invaluable support, along with the other sponsors and supporters who got behind us, had got us to the start line, we were still working on a tight budget; the costs wouldn't stop until we reached Hawaii and shipped *Bo* home. We had barely a week until the race began. Every moment of spare time was spent working on the boat and her equipment. Packing and repacking, fixing equipment that wasn't working and fitting new kit. It was a tense time.

Coincidentally, Nat had been working in San Francisco in the weeks leading up to our arrival in her capacity as an events manager. So as soon as her contract finished, she drove down to Monterey to help us out. As well as being fantastic to see her, it was a vital help. Three sets of hands made all the difference getting the last-minute jobs done. It took some of the pressure off and allowed it to become a more enjoyable experience for all three of us.

We were always going to make the start date, but when news came that the weather forecast was bad, I was relieved they'd decided to delay the start by four days. We were meant to leave on 2 June and it was put back to the 6th. It gave us a little more time to fix some of the kit that was giving us problems. The autopilot system on the rudder, which I'd always had my doubts about, was not performing properly, and some of the electronics were problematic. In an ideal world I'd have replaced everything, but the budget had never allowed for that. Fortunately, Justin Aitken was working for Chris Martin in Monterey, helping the teams with the last-minute equipment issues like these.

Justin's an excellent boat builder and an accomplished ocean rower. We'd competed in the same Atlantic rowing race in 2005 and were old friends. I ran a couple of the problems past him and, typically, he found solutions and promptly sorted them for me. It was a big help. Time was tight but everything was steadily falling into place.

There was one extra thing we hadn't anticipated. Just before we'd flown out, Sparky had been to see his doctor. A couple of times when he'd been training on the rowing machine he found he'd become breathless, and he'd wanted to make sure it was nothing serious. He had a series of blood tests which alarmingly suggested he may have the early symptoms of angina. He'd need an angiogram to confirm the extent of the problem, but there was no way he could have one before we were due to leave.

He'd told me just prior to our departure to the US, and, of course, I immediately assumed he wouldn't be able to take part.

'No,' Sparky said, 'I've spoken to my doctor. It's manageable. We can take precautions for the row.'

'But people die from angina,' I said.

'Mate, if I'm going to die from angina, I'd rather it happen trying to row the Pacific than sat in the chair at home,' he replied. The fact that he was far less likely to have an attack and die sitting in the chair back home as opposed to if he was rowing the Pacific didn't come into his thinking.

Sparky eventually got the signed go-ahead from his doctor before we left, on the condition that the race medical authorities cleared it before we set off on the row.

So now we had a worrying meeting with Chris and with Aeynor Sawyer, the race doctor in Monterey, to discuss the problem and confirm the measures we'd take to deal with any potential problem during the race. It was a nervous time as Sparky outlined his symptoms and his UK doctors' evaluation of his condition, while Aeynor analysed the potential risks Sparky might be taking and if acceptable measures could be put in place to negate them. Sparky and I were both aware as we sat across the table from Chris and Aeynor that our race could be about to come to an end, even before it started.

Although both trying our best to look unconcerned, we breathed a huge sigh of relief when a solution was agreed upon and Sparky was given the green light to participate. We would take a healthy supply of nitroglycerine spray, which we would both carry on our bodies, so any attack could be addressed immediately with a squirt of the drug under Sparky's tongue.

It appeared even a dodgy heart wasn't going to stop us rowing the Pacific Ocean.

CHAPTER 22

SPARKY THE OAR SLAYER

Appropriately enough, our own D-Day, the delayed race start, came on the 6 June 2018, the seventy-fourth anniversary of the considerably more significant original D-Day, when allied forces stormed the beaches of Normandy in 1944. The race fleet, seven strong on our arrival in California, was reduced to five by the time we departed. There were two fours (one all-male crew, one all-female), an all-female trio, and two pairs boats, both male crews, one of which comprised of Sparky and me, the oldest competitors in the race.

When we rowed out of the harbour towards the official starting point, I was relieved to finally be setting off, but that sense of relief came with anxiety and a tinge of regret. The timeframe and tight budget had dominated the build-up, and not in a good way. Initially the plan had been to refit and improve *Bo*. But we were only able to get her back to where she was a decade previously. In fact, in some ways, I felt she was less well-equipped. I had hoped that we might challenge the record crossing for a pair, which was fifty-six days. As we left Monterey Bay behind, I doubted that was possible.

Almost all the improvements and modifications I'd planned were dropped because of cost. We made do with equipment which was old but functioning. New, lighter rowing seats and rails, and, crucially, a much-improved steering system, were simply too expensive.

Bo was well built, safe and as strong as ever. Twenty-one feet long, six feet at her widest point, she was a totally self-sufficient and proven ocean rowing boat. Solar rechargeable batteries provided her power and a built-in water maker created ample fresh water for the duration of any voyage. A small watertight cabin at the rear gave us somewhere to sleep between our two hour alternate shifts at the oars and a safe place to retreat to when storms hit. With fourteen watertight compartments along the length of her hull, where our food for the voyage was stored, she was effectively unsinkable. An additional fifty kilos of lead, which I built into her keel, made her especially resistant to capsize and even more likely to self-right if she ever did go over. *Bo* was the best ocean rowing boat in the world when I built her for the North Pacific row in 2009, and even now, almost a decade later, she was still a fantastic boat. I couldn't help feeling, though, that we'd missed an opportunity to make her better, more efficient and potentially competitive. As much as I realised it was all about finishing, there was a part of me that felt this race was winnable. If we won, it would have given Sparky an even greater platform to inspire people with his story, which would add value to what we were trying to achieve beyond simply rowing the Pacific. I had no idea then just how grateful I would eventually be simply to finish the Great Pacific Race.

My concerns about what might have been were irrelevant as we reached the imaginary starting line between two buoys just outside the harbour. All that mattered now was how two men in a twenty-one-foot rowing boat, one of them blind, both with more years gone than they could reasonably anticipate to come, coped with all the Pacific Ocean chose to throw at them in the months and miles ahead. There are few people in the world with more experience in ocean rowing boats than me, but even I would be surprised at just how much that would prove to be.

The first few hours, unsurprisingly, were a tough initiation into the race, but a helpful one. We departed at 5 p.m. to take advantage of the strong south-easterly land breeze which generally sets in at the end of the day in the bay, as the land cools and the wind sweeps down from the hills and out to sea. The waves were choppy but manageable and we were able to hold a course just north of west, out and away from Monterey Bay. We took it as a good omen when several whales surfaced for air near us as we left Point Pinos Lighthouse, the mark on the southernmost headland of the bay behind, and entered the Pacific Ocean.

Twelve hours later that helpful south-easterly land breeze had backed all the way around to an unhelpful north-westerly. It didn't stop us completely, but it slowed our speed and pushed us south as we tried to make progress west. Within the next twenty-four hours, this unhelpful wind built to near gale force. The waves took on the fierce granite complexion I'd seen so many times before as they grew steadily with the increasing wind speeds. The wind chill matched the bitterly cold sea temperature and ominously threatening slate grey clouds stretched past every horizon.

'I don't seem to remember you mentioning this in your description of the Pacific in The Coach House, Mick,' Sparky shouted above the noise of the wind as we swapped over at the end of his two-hour shift.

We were both dressed in our full anti-foul gear, as we had been since departure. We were also both cold and soaking wet as a result of the constant hits we were taking from the large waves regularly washing over us. Again, as we had been since departure.

'It'll get better every day,' I assured him, laughing.

I said that every day from the day we left. It didn't. Neither of us realised it then, but it would be several weeks before it got any better at all, and before then it was going to get a lot worse.

Sparky was incredible from day one. His refusal to be limited by his disability, as well as being utterly inspirational to witness, meant there were many times I'd have to remind myself he was

149

blind. We'd been through every locker and container in the boat beforehand together so he could memorise where everything was, creating his mind map, as he called it. The only thing he couldn't do was cook.

Sparky insisted as a result that other regular jobs on board would be his sole responsibility. Servicing the bearings and replacing the wheels on the rowing seats was one of the jobs he eagerly took on. A messy and fiddly job on dry land, this was even more so on the unstable deck of an ocean rowing boat.

We fell easily into the two hours on, two hours off rowing routine, and despite the bitterly cold and wet conditions, we were rising to the challenge as I knew we would. It was just like being back in the marines again. Long hours, lousy pay, cold, wet, little sleep and looking forwards to a beer when it was all over. *Exactly* like being in the marines again.

After the start, our small race fleet had slowly progressed along their own individually chosen headings and the distances between us all had quickly increased. Within hours of setting off each team soon found themselves completely alone on a vast ocean, with the distant silhouette of land rapidly disappearing behind them and none of their competitors in sight. The significance of the race we'd all spent so much time and effort preparing for faded slowly along with the North American continent, as the only real adversary any of us faced took centre stage: the Pacific Ocean.

For almost a week we battled across seemingly never-ending north or north-westerly winds. It made for painfully slow and constantly cold and wet progress towards our next goal, the distant easterly trade winds, supposedly just a couple of hundred miles away, which should help push us towards Honolulu. But right now the winds pushed us further south, steadily adding extra miles to our journey. We'd briefly deployed the parachute anchor a couple of times at night just to ride out the really big seas, but generally we'd coped well and were making constant, albeit slow, progress.

I'd been amazed at how Sparky had adapted. The autopilot system installed to help him steer simply couldn't cope with the conditions we were facing, so we rapidly gave up on that. I'd never had much faith in it. Instead, Sparky had two audio compasses which emitted corrective beeps to help prevent him straying off course. They too had their limitations, however, particularly in strong winds and heavy seas.

Fortunately, we realised very early on that Sparky could make out the shape of the large Union flag we had flying above the port side of the cabin in his peripheral vision. Even at night, with the navigation light on, he could pick up its shape and, by virtue of that, he knew which direction the wind was blowing. So long as the wind didn't change direction, that meant the flag became a reference point for Sparky as to whether he was on course or not.

After that discovery, every handover began with me directing Sparky on to the course he needed to be rowing and then him equating that course with the shape of the flag flying in the wind. If he kept the flag flying in that direction for his two-hour watch, he was pretty much on course. It was by no means flawless, but it worked.

I encouraged Sparky to recognise where the wind was blowing on his face and how and where the waves were striking the boat to help develop his sense of position and course too. It was going back to the basics of sailing by touch and feel rather than by technology, and, as ever, Sparky rose to the challenge.

A week into the row and the weather hadn't let up. The Pacific Ocean off California in June reminded me more of the North Sea off Grimsby in October. I hadn't seen more than a glimmer of blue sky since the start, let alone felt the sun on my face. Strong winds created an intimidatingly angry rolling sea that resembled fluid fields of jagged rocks, and bitterly cold temperatures left us living in our foul-weather gear.

The wind continued to blow from the north, which meant we could row, but it left us beam on to the waves. It's a nasty situation in a rowing boat for a normally sighted person, but for a visually impaired rower who couldn't see the waves coming it was potentially lethal. Despite this, Sparky was coping brilliantly and happily maintained his end of the brutal two hours on two hours off rowing routine. Our progress was slow but we were making our way west. We just needed to keep going.

On 13 June, the day after the fourth birthday I'd celebrated rowing across the Pacific, the weather deteriorated even further. The wind became stronger and it backed more to the west, making progress even more painfully slow and creating increasingly large and intimidating seas. I knew that this would be just the kind of weather in which we could make ground on the other less-experienced teams, who'd most likely use their para anchors to ride out the weather. I also knew how increasingly exposed we were to potential capsize, particularly for Sparky, who simply wouldn't see a big breaking wave coming.

As the dusk fell and darkness engulfed us, I handed over to Sparky. I could already see how increasingly formidable the conditions were becoming.

'I think we're going to need to put the para anchor in soon, mate, just to be on the safe side.'

'Why? It's not that bad yet, is it?' Sparky responded.

'It's getting that way, mate. Won't be much longer at this rate before we need to put it in. Are you happy to carry on for now?'

'Yeah, I'm fine, mate.'

'Well so long as you're OK. If you feel it pick up any more, give me a shout and we'll put the para anchor in.'

Ironically, the strong north-west winds made maintaining a course easier for Sparky, as it blew the flag at almost right angles across the boat, making it clearer for him to make out. *Bo* was a great sea boat, so once the rudder and her trim was set, she carved a reliable course across the waves.

Exhausted, I fell into a deep sleep as soon as I climbed back into the tiny cabin at the stern of the boat, leaving Sparky to it. Crawling out on deck less than two hours later for my next shift at the oars, I knew immediately things had got worse. The wind was gusting at more than thirty-five knots now and the waves had grown larger and angrier.

'Mate, this has picked up a bit. You should have called me. I reckon we need to put the para anchor in now,' I shouted over the wind.

'Well,' Sparky replied in indignation, 'if I can row in this, you should be all right, shouldn't you?'

'Yeah, I suppose you might have a point there, mate,' I answered, smiling.

Two hours later Sparky emerged once more from the cabin and closed the hatch behind him.

'Are you sure you're happy to row in this, Sparky?'

'I'm clipped on, so I'll be fine.' He gestured to the harness around his shoulders which he constantly had attached to the boat when on deck.

The fact that Sparky had coped so well with the constant bad weather and miserable conditions we'd been battling since starting the race had served to lull me into a false sense of security. His now fearless approach towards the building storm only increased that effect. He so relentlessly refused to give in to his disability it became infectious. Not for the first time, and certainly not for the last time on that voyage, I was almost disregarding the fact that Sparky couldn't see. He had limitations I wasn't taking into account because he was coping with them so well.

He'd had a point earlier when he said I should be able to row on in conditions that he could cope with. This was not just because I had my sight, but also because of my rowing experience. But there still had to be a cut-off point for him and for us as a team in bad weather. It was my job to decide when that was. Because Sparky was so remarkable at dealing with his condition in any environment, I'd failed to do that job. I'd failed to recognise we'd crossed that safe cut-off point. We should have stopped rowing no later than that shift change over and put the parachute anchor in. My failure to make that decision would have almost fatal consequences.

I crawled into the cabin, the only lights visible tiny red and green circuit and power lights on various instruments on the control panels fitted into the bulkhead either side of the main hatch. I reached into my pocket for a protein bar to eat before sleeping. I took a single bite before *Bo* was hit by what seemed like a freight train. There was what felt and sounded like an explosion as hundreds of tons of water hit the boat and threw her on her side. She was hit by and buried under a monster wave which seemed to smash over us for a lifetime. The power failed and I remember hearing *Bo* cracking and creaking under the impact. I'm not certain another ocean rowing boat would have remained intact. A few moments later an even bigger wave hurtled into us, burying us again under tonnes of tumbling water.

Bo began to fight back against this mountain of water, stubbornly refusing to capsize and steadily rolling upright again. It was a miracle she had remained in one piece. The power flickered back into life inside the cabin, another stroke of luck.

Most important, though, was Sparky OK?

I rushed out of the cabin, sealing the hatch behind me against any further hits as I stepped carefully into the cockpit. It was turmoil on deck, understandably, but I was hugely relieved to see

Sparky still on board and connected to the boat. He was laid out where he'd obviously been thrown, shaken but seemingly OK.

I'd later discover he'd been swept off his seat by the first wave that had broadsided us. He'd been fully submerged as *Bo* was knocked onto her starboard beam and then hit again by the second wave. Fortunately, his harness had kept him attached to the boat and as *Bo* had begun to self-right, he said, 'She just scooped me up out of the water, dragging me back on board.'

He'd already become fond of *Bo*, as everyone does when they get to know her. Now he was besotted with her. She'd saved his life.

I saw that, even laid as he was in the scuppers to the side of the rowing position on the deck, he still held in his hands two halves of the oars he'd been rowing with. They'd both been snapped completely in half when the wave hit. He held them up in front of him, indicating how, despite the damage, he'd not let go.

'You do realise we're going to have to pay for them,' I said dryly.

He looked at me open mouthed, working out if I was joking or not. I was. We *were* going to have to pay for them at some point, but it was a joke. I was overjoyed and relieved he was still on the boat. That was all that mattered. If his harness had failed and he'd been separated from *Bo*, I've no doubt that in the dark and in those conditions he would have died. I'd never have been able to find him and he wouldn't have been able to see the boat to get back to it, even if he were able. It was a ferocious hit, one of the biggest, if not the biggest, I've ever experienced on an ocean rowing boat, and we'd luckily survived.

'Are you sure you're OK, mate?' I asked, taking the remnants of the two snapped oars from him and helping him up.

'Yeah, yeah, I'm good, nothing broken, apart from the oars. A bit shook up, but I'm OK.'

'OK to carry on rowing?' I asked, straight-faced.

There was a pause as Sparky positioned himself back on the rowing seat.

'Yeeesss?' he asked, rather than stated, slowly and rather unconvincingly. Nooo! I think he wanted to say, but I admired his determination.

I laughed. 'Forget it, mate. We'll stick the para anchor in and get some rest while this settles down.'

CHAPTER 23

WE'RE OUT OF THE RACE

Having survived the knockdown and then riding out the remainder of the storm on the para anchor, we set off again with renewed vigour later that day. An unexpected break from the painfully relentless rowing routine was always gratefully received. But release from the claustrophobic confines of the cabin, where we were both locked inside together for several hours, was equally welcome. The milder conditions and slightly warmer temperatures which greeted us on deck made that release even more pleasant. Perhaps today was finally going to be a better day.

Unfortunately, it wasn't. The next two weeks would prove to be a sequence of false dawns, bad news and unexpected setbacks. The milder conditions proved to be the first false dawn. By nightfall the wind had backed all the way around towards the west again, blowing almost directly onto the nose of our boat. It was slowly building in strength and it was once again bitterly cold.

The sea took on the constitution of liquid cement. The little distance we made against the conditions was heartbreakingly disproportionate to the gargantuan effort we were putting in to achieve it. By dawn the next day when the wind finally became too strong to counter, exhausted and despondent we redeployed the parachute anchor and collapsed into the cabin once more.

News from the race headquarters was even more alarming. Our rivals in the pairs race had been capsized in the heavy winds which had knocked us down and made short work of Sparky's oars. Despite their boat self-righting successfully, one of the guys had been on deck and had developed hypothermia. Reluctantly, they'd decided to call for rescue when his symptoms failed to improve.

They were an experienced and a very competent team who'd recently rowed the Atlantic together – Mike Matson and Brian Krauskopf. We'd got to know them quite well during the build-up in Monterey. It was a shock they were out of the race so soon – I had them down as the likely winners. We were disappointed for them but at the same time relieved they were both OK.

'Look on the bright side, Sparky,' I said dryly, after I relayed the news. 'We're first in class now, mate.'

He shook his head in mock disdain.

A second boat was rescued a couple of days later. Apparently, the female fours team, in *Ripple Effect*, had deployed the parachute anchor when the storm hit and had been badly battered by the winds and waves for several days. Their boat design, similar to Mike and Brian's pairs boat, had a shallow keel and a large forward cabin. It was built for speed in front of following steady trade winds, not stability riding out storms. Sea sickness had become debilitating for some of the crew, so they called for rescue.

Bo and the other two remaining boats in the race were classic designs, lower profile with deeper, more angular drafts, and therefore more purchase on the water. They coped far better with the unexpectedly rough weather and the extended periods on the para anchor.

The loss of two boats little more than a week into the race confirmed just how tough the conditions had been, and probably helped to put into perspective our own trials and tribulations. Everybody was having a tough time. It was just a matter of keeping going.

'Well,' Sparky said to me, after I told him about the second boats rescue, 'look on the bright side, mate. We're guaranteed first in class and at least third overall now.'

It was my turn to shake my head.

'Only if we finish, mate,' I replied. 'Only if we finish.'

We returned to the oars when the wind allowed and continued to push west whenever we were able during the following days. The winds continued to force us further south than we wished. We were taking the longer route to Hawaii, whether we liked it or not. Potentially helpful trade winds were by now very close, but still agonisingly just out of reach.

The remaining fours team, Uniting Nations on board *Danielle*, however, had been able to punch west. Rowing three at a time almost around the clock, a supreme effort, they'd eventually escaped the winds that were hampering our progress. They could now row a direct course to Honolulu with the bonus of steady and helpful trade winds filling in behind them.

Barring unforeseen injury or equipment failure, that fantastic effort would win the race for them. Neither we nor the three girls in Pacific Terrific onboard *Isabelle*, the third boat still in the race, were in a position to catch them now. We were both still losing distance south as we attempted to row west. *Danielle*, on the other hand, was heading directly towards Hawaii. Every hour at the oars dragged them further away from us and closer to the finish line.

Sparky and I were holding on to second place at the time, although only a few miles separated us from Pacific Terrific. Having a rival in relatively close proximity fuelled our competitive streak and helped ensure we maintained the gruelling rowing routine we'd embarked on at departure. Two hours on, two hours off, around the clock. Only severe weather occasionally interrupted that relentless schedule. It's an exhausting routine and probably explains why, midway through the third week, Sparky had a small accident which had a massive impact on me.

There's a procedure on board ocean rowing boats which Chris Martin and I had christened The Midnight Shuffle. It's a technique to safely change places on a rowing boat at night in rough seas. Both crew members face each other directly along the length of the deck, one at the rowing position, one in front of the cabin, each holding the grab lines which run waist height from the aft cabin to the forward cabin, either side of the boat. Crouching like underfed sumo wrestlers they then, on an agreed signal, move symmetrically clockwise, until both crew members have swapped positions. If done correctly it takes seconds, keeps the boat stable and the crew safe from injury or the threat of being washed overboard.

Sadly, almost a decade later, Sparky and I managed to make our version of that slick procedure more often resemble an elderly, naked, slow-motion version of Twister. On one particularly fatigued occasion I remember replacing Sparky at the oars. We set ourselves up facing one another and prepared to move on the agreed signal, when I shouted 'Now!' I moved immediately. Sparky, unfortunately, delayed. It wasn't a major problem to begin with, it just caused *Bo* to heel a little over to one side. A split-second later Sparky stumbled forwards trying to make up for his hesitation and, as he passed me in the dark, I heard a dull thud and a pain-filled moan.

Without looking back, I shouted, 'Please tell me that was your toe, not your head, mate!'

'It was my fucking nose,' he replied, his voice now muffled by his hands cupping his face.

He'd missed his footing as we passed and, off balance from the boat heeling, he'd fallen forwards. He'd lost his grip on the line he'd been holding and, desperately trying to grab it again, the next thing he knew his nose had smashed into the corner of the cabin roof.

I turned to see him sitting outside the main hatch, clutching his now battered and bleeding face.

'How many times am I going to break my fucking nose?'

This was obviously not a first.

I tried not to laugh despite the painfully comic circumstances. I realised he was in considerable pain and it was one more discomfort for him to put up with on the boat. Despite the darkness, I could see there was a lot of blood and his already battered nose did look, on closer inspection, even more out of shape than normal.

Less than twelve hours later, as a result of that almost laughable accident, I glimpsed for the first time the true enormity of what I'd asked of Steve Sparkes, and at the same time I also finally grasped the enormous courage he possessed.

The bleeding had stopped fairly quickly but it became apparent the next morning that there was a lot of swelling on and around his nose, with two vivid black eyes forming. At the time, this only added to the comic value of the whole episode. I noticed Steve's mood had changed, though. For the first time during the whole trip he seemed distant, subdued and more than a little anxious.

'Are you OK, mate?' I asked during one of our changeovers.

'It's nothing. I'm just a bit worried about my eyes. The swelling is affecting my peripheral vision. I can't even make out shapes properly now. I'm a bit worried about what I've done. If I get an infection out here, I could lose what's left of my eyesight. I'll be completely blind.'

It hit me like a hammer blow. Although Sparky was registered blind, that small percentage of peripheral vision which he still retained dramatically contributed to his quality of life. Combined with his relentless positivity and can-do attitude, it allowed him a level of independence which, if he lost it, would be disastrous.

He'd lost most of his sight once and now he had a very real concern that he could, in effect, lose it once again.

I felt the crushing emotional impact of having put him in the position where that could happen. I realised yet again how I'd been so in awe of how well Sparky coped with his condition, I'd become, ironically enough, blind to the challenges and issues he faced every day of his life. Anyone else would have retreated into a bubble of self-protection. Sparky had done the reverse. He'd enthusiastically placed himself in one of the most hostile and threat-rich environments anyone could imagine, let alone a visually impaired person.

Despite that shattering realisation, I still had no regrets asking Sparky to come on the row. Quite the opposite, as his attitude to his disability served only to reconfirm to me that he was uniquely suited to successfully completing the voyage.

I had, though, become truly aware for the first time of the potentially devastating personal consequences Sparky was facing rowing an ocean, the unique risks he was taking. He, of course, had been aware of them from the moment I suggested it. He lived with that realisation every day of his life. What made Sparky remarkable was that he didn't use those consequences as an excuse to shy away from life. In fact, he used them as an excuse to embrace it, to overcome the challenges in front of him and use each of those victories to conquer the disability which had never come close to defeating him. Rowing the Pacific was just Sparky once again demonstrating his blindness hadn't beaten him. His nose may have been fragile, but he had the heart and the courage of a lion.

Much to my relief, and Sparky's, the damage to his peripheral vision proved temporary. He slowly recovered as the swelling around his nose eventually subsided over the following days. The weather conditions, however, weren't so amenable.

A few days after Sparky broke his nose, we had our first flat calm day. Not a breath of wind. Never a great scenario on an ocean rowing boat, and without the helpful outline of our Union flag fluttering in the breeze, Sparky now had no reference points to steer a course from. He fell back completely on his audio compass. For a while this worked well, but we soon discovered that when night settled in the solar rechargeable batteries rapidly lost power, leaving the unit dead until sunrise.

When we could see the moon, he used that as a reference, and likewise the sun during the day. This was vital, because the auto pilot never worked effectively and the audio compasses eventually fell apart before we were halfway across.

But on the nights when there was no breeze and no moon, Sparky had no option other than to stop rowing for much of the time during his night shifts. It was incredibly frustrating, especially for Sparky on deck. These were needlessly lost miles which were slipping away from us, undermining all our hard work. Once more it came down to the fundamental problem we'd battled throughout the project. We hadn't had the funding to purchase the kit we needed to be as effective as possible on the row. It would be a constant issue. It remained to be seen if it would eventually prove fatal to our hopes.

As frustrating as those becalmed miles were, much worse was to come. We'd noticed when replacing the first set of oars destroyed in the storm that one of the two remaining spare sets was slightly shorter than the other. Hardly perceptible stowed on deck, but, when in the rowing gates, the difference in power and output was alarming. They felt almost like toy oars in comparison. They'd been kindly loaned to us by my friend and fellow ocean rower Charlie Martell, owner of the *Black Pig*, just days before *Bo* was shipped. I hadn't realised his boat was a slightly narrower design than ours and, consequently, his oars didn't need to be quite as long. We'd initially replaced the first broken set with them only to discover they were massively underpowered, and hurriedly replaced them with the other spare set.

All of the three sets of oars we'd taken on board were the same specialist make, Xcel Ocean, which I'd used successfully many times before and would recommend for any ocean row. However, two of the sets, the ones which had come with *Bo*, were old, veterans of several crossings, and bore all the resulting wear and tear. The third set were too short. With one set gone, we were now effectively on our last effective set of oars on the boat. To make matters worse, on several occasions the collars which locked that set into the rowing gates had fallen apart due to their age. This left the oars vulnerable to slipping out of the gate. It wasn't a big deal when it happened to me, but with Sparky's lack of vision it could be disastrous. We could easily lose one of the oars.

We were ultra-cautious with this second set of oars. I constantly checked on the collars to head off any failure which could see us losing one over the side. When the wind picked up we now looked to deploy the para anchor sooner than normal, to avoid another incident where we could snap an oar.

As we entered the fourth week of the row, disaster inevitably struck. It was just before dusk and I'd been rowing in choppy seas with a strong breeze. The light was beginning to fade on another grey, cold day on the Pacific. I was wearing my heavy jacket to ward off the cold and the waves. It was as well I did. I'm certain I would have died that night if I hadn't.

Sparky and I had just swapped places, with him taking over on the oars and I heading towards the cabin for a couple of hours' sleep. Sparky had released the oars which had been secured across the boat but unfortunately, by mistake, had let them sit loose in the gates, the ends of the oars hanging in the water. It was something we avoided doing at all costs as it left the blade vulnerable to being broken by an unexpected wave and, with the unreliable collars securing them, potentially slipping overboard.

We were both tired. Sparky had just woken up and he hadn't realised that when he untied the blades they had slipped over the side, secured only by their collars in the gates. Normally even this wouldn't have been a major problem, but at that moment the collar on the starboard oar came apart and completely separated from the shaft. The blade fired, silently, torpedo-like, out of the gate into the ocean, the broken collars dropping uselessly to the deck. Sparky obviously couldn't see it and only realised there was a problem when he reached for where he thought the blade should be.

'One of my oars is gone!' he shouted suddenly.

I turned, startled. 'What do you mean?'

Looking down I could see an empty rowing gate and the remains of the collar on the deck. No more than three or four feet from the side of the boat the shaft of the blade was in the water. The wind was blowing strongly, pushing us steadily further and further from the irreplaceable oar.

I jumped on the side of the boat and hanging on to the safety lines with one hand and stretching out as far as I could, I tried desperately to scoop it back using my foot. It was agonisingly just out of reach. My first instinct was to dive in after the oar and recover it. The fact that I'd been wearing my heavy jacket made that impossible. That delay while I tried to stretch out from the boat and reach the blade probably saved my life. Having failed to drag it back towards us, I started to strip off the jacket. Sparky was doing all he could with the remaining oar to stop us drifting away.

'What are you going to do?' he shouted.

'I'm going in after it,' I shouted back.

'Don't be stupid, mate, you won't get back on board in this wind,' he cried.

It stopped me in my tracks. He was right. The boat was already several yards away from the blade and I was struggling to keep it in sight. The waves were large enough that it was disappearing into each trough. To make matters worse, the wind was blowing us away from the oar at an alarmingly swift rate. There was little Sparky could do with just the one remaining oar to stop that.

The light was fading rapidly. There was an almost primeval threat to the situation developing which I could sense physically. I'd been on the verge of making a foolish and what I'm sure would have been fatal mistake diving overboard to recover the lost blade. I felt a chill move down my spine as I watched for just a few seconds more as the blade disappeared completely from sight and the twilight heralding the coming night consumed us. If I'd been in the ocean, I have no doubt I would not have made it back to the boat, with or without the precious oar.

Just as importantly, my actions could have created a life-threatening emergency for Sparky. If I'd been lost at sea he'd have been left to cope alone on the boat. We'd discussed this 'unlikely' possibility in the preparation for the race and Sparky was competent and more than familiar with all the life-saving devices on board in an emergency. There's no question, though, it was a situation which could have put his life in very real jeopardy. I had to remind myself that my responsibility wasn't to reach Hawaii quickly, my only responsibility was to ensure Sparky arrived safely.

I knew from the moment the oar disappeared our race was over. It was now all about just getting to the finish line.

Without thinking, I spat out, 'Well that's just added another two weeks to the trip.'

I could sense Sparky's despondency at my comment.

'Well, maybe not two weeks, maybe just a couple of extra days,' I lied, trying to remain positive for both our sakes.

I believe there are times in all our lives when the Grim Reaper swoops close by, offering a hand for the foolish to grasp, waiting for a stupid or poor decision to take advantage of or a stroke of bad luck that might allow him to claim us. I have absolutely no doubt, for me, that evening was one such time. There was an ominous sense of foreboding about the whole episode, and if death creates an aura it rapidly descended upon events as they escalated. In the aftermath of losing the oar, which was a disaster in terms of us completing the row quickly, if at all, my only emotion was fear. Not fear we wouldn't reach Hawaii, but fear of how narrowly I'd escaped a lingering, cold and lonely death in the Pacific Ocean and how narrowly I'd escaped potentially condemning my friend to the same fate.

CHAPTER 24

BLIND VISION

The overwhelming disappointment of losing the third oar was tempered by my lucky escape trying to recover it. It was a setback, but it could easily have been much worse. We could still reach Hawaii. It would take longer for sure, but there was no reason we couldn't successfully complete the voyage. I'd have to encourage Sparky the Oar Slayer to be a little less wasteful with the remaining set of blades, but we were still on track to reach the finish line. Any hopes of giving the three girls on *Isabelle* a race into Honolulu had pretty much disappeared – they were ahead of us now in second place and making great progress. We'd do our best to give them a race, but, if nothing else, hopefully we could at least arrive in time to have a beer with them in Honolulu.

The days which immediately followed the dramatic loss of the third oar did nothing to lighten our mood. Although temperatures were milder, it was still overcast, grey and sunless. Most frustratingly, the wind, although lighter, continued to blow relentlessly from the north. Progress was slow and hard-earned. We were both becoming exhausted physically and mentally. The knowledge that every day's mileage was now less than it would have been if we hadn't lost the third oar only added to that exhaustion.

To make matters worse, we heard that the football World Cup had started back home and England, for once, were playing well.

'If I'm out here with you when England finally manage to win the World Cup again I'm going to be really pissed off, Mick,' Sparky said slowly, when I gave him the news England had qualified from their group for the knockout stages.

'What's the chances of that happening, mate?' I replied, laughing.

On 3 July, England beat Columbia 5–4 on penalties to reach the quarter finals. Their chances were getting stronger.

Our luck appeared to be changing, too. The wind, although still light, had finally come around to just east of north, and although not quite the easterly trade winds we were eagerly anticipating, it was finally offering us some gentle assistance towards our destination. Despite this long overdue good fortune, progress continued to be slow and exhausting and it started to take its toll on the pair of us physically.

I was the first to feel the strain as our bodies dealt with the punishing regime we were employing. By 5 July my right shoulder was in agony. It had steadily become worse since we lost the third oar, although I don't believe the events were connected. I was always reluctant to use medication unless absolutely necessary at sea, but eventually I had no choice but to raid the medical supplies for a solution. Ibuprofen should do the trick, I figured. It would almost certainly be inflammation of the tissue around my shoulder joint caused by the relentless workload. Within an hour of taking the first tablet my shoulder pain was gone. I could row without pain and, just as importantly, I could sleep without it. I kicked myself for not taking it sooner. I'd been in pain needlessly for almost a week by then.

A day or so later we realised our easterly winds weren't a taste of things to come. They were just another false dawn. Early in the morning the wind began to back slowly to the north once more while steadily increasing in strength. By night we found ourselves battling an unhelpful wind and sea yet again. It reduced our speed and it forced us further and further south, adding extra unwanted miles to our voyage.

* * *

A particularly significant day for me personally was 8 July. It is the anniversary of my father's death. I had been rowing across the North Pacific with Chris Martin when my dad passed away. Nine years later, to be rowing on the Pacific once more only added to the poignancy of the date.

In 2009, I'd reacted to the news, at least initially, by throwing myself completely into the rowing, as I thought my dad would have expected. I simply battled through it. In effect, all I did was set myself on a course for physical and emotional exhaustion and ultimately failure. I was rowing every two hours but rarely sleeping in between. When I did sleep I woke once again to the agonising realisation that my dad had died. I seldom spoke and was slowly being consumed by the grief and guilt I wasn't willing to acknowledge. I can only imagine how it must have seemed to Chris, trapped on the boat with me. Fortunately, in the most unlikely of ways, the weather came to my rescue.

The wind, as it often did on the North Pacific, swung round to the east, the direction we were heading. It wasn't particularly strong, but strong enough to put a stop to our rowing. We deployed the parachute anchor and waited for the weather to change. It was forecast to be over a week before we would be able to make progress again.

At the time I'd thought it would destroy me. The lack of progress towards our goal turning the voyage into what I considered a prison sentence. As it turned out, it was precisely what I needed. It meant I was no longer able to destroy myself at the oars, I was no longer exhausted and I was able to finally rest properly, and as a result had time to think clearly and acknowledge what had happened. Eventually, I realised in many ways I'd been blessed. I was able to spend each day on the para anchor simply remembering my dad and the experiences we'd shared. Few people have that opportunity when they're bereaved, as there's just too much to arrange and sort out when someone close to you dies. The remembering comes later when the chaos of coping with an unexpected death has settled down.

I remember vividly the day of my father's funeral, although it was the middle of the night for me out on the Pacific. *Bo* was still on the parachute anchor and was I laid on her deck looking up at a night sky packed full of distant galaxies with their myriad stars. I don't think I'd ever truly recognised the universe's awe-inspiring beauty before. For several hours I lay staring into that infinite spectacle, remembering my dad and coming to terms with my loss. There's nothing quite like appreciating your place in the universe to put things in perspective. It was one of many lessons I learned rowing the North Pacific, and it helped to get me back on track mentally to complete our record-breaking row into San Francisco. It was a lesson that would also help when I returned to row the Pacific again with Sparky.

As we prepared ourselves for one more battle against the conditions, the news came through that England had beaten Sweden two-nil in their World Cup quarterfinal. They were now one just game away from a World Cup final.

'The gods are laughing at us, Mick, you do realise that, don't you?' Sparky said disconsolately when I told him.

We'd been battling the Pacific Ocean for over a month now, and it had been an increasingly tough battle. It wasn't lost on me that, if I was finding it tough going, how the hell was Sparky finding it?

It was not the experience I'd expected and not the experience I'd promised him. It had been a cold, wet and frighteningly hostile introduction to ocean rowing for Sparky. After a month at sea I had logged only four days where we even saw a glimpse of the sun and blue skies, let alone had a sunny day. The remainder of our days were dominated by oppressive grey cloud cover either side of the strong winds and storms that had frequently battered us.

As night fell on 8 July, I realised it was the first night there wasn't a cloud in the sky. The universe in all its glory was on display for the first time. It was a sight I'd seen from the deck of an ocean rowing boat hundreds of times before, but one that had never lost its impact.

'Sparky, if I turned off the navigation light, would you be able to see any of the stars with your peripheral vision?' I asked.

'It's effectively my night vision that's left so I should be able to. Why?'

I retreated to the cabin and switched off our single white navigation light, which was fitted on a pole above the forward cabin. It left Sparky alone on an unlit rowing deck, his only illumination a spectacular moonless universe which stretched out all around him, filling a cloudless sky.

I could see his silhouette against the stars as he tilted his head back to allow his vision to adjust and take in this incredible sight. There was not one bit of light pollution. This was the cosmos at its purest, in all its breath-taking beauty. Sparky, a man registered blind, was now seeing a view of the universe few people on the surface of the planet had ever or would ever see in their lives. Whatever the hardships of the previous month at sea, for the first time I felt it was becoming worth it. For the first time Sparky was getting something special from this experience. Something he deserved and something he'd earned.

CHAPTER 25

IN SICKNESS AND IN HEALTH

The enormous sense of pride I took from seeing Sparky silhouetted against that incredible star-filled night, taking in such a unique view of the universe, was short lived. Unhelpfully, I'd promptly fallen asleep in the cabin, leaving Sparky outside in the darkness. As a result, he had no way to see the flag he used to steer a course by when he wanted to start rowing again.

Twenty minutes later I awoke from a deep sleep, more akin to a coma, to Sparky's shouts of, 'Mick! Turn the navigation light back on, you knob! I can't see which way to row!'

Our fortunes began to decline in tandem with the England football team's. They stumbled to a 2–1 defeat against Croatia despite a mouth-watering contest against the hosts, France, awaiting them in the final. For Sparky, I think in some ways that may have been a relief. I'm not sure he'd have ever forgiven himself, or me, if he'd missed England in a World Cup final. Fortunately, we never had to find out.

With the distant disappointment of our nation's footballing exploits came more pertinent, personal disappointments. The northerly winds which had plagued us almost constantly since departure were still hampering our progress west. To make matters worse they were picking up to near gale-force strength once again. We'd fallen into such a relentless routine of battling across these conditions that it hadn't occurred to me that Sparky might be struggling. Primarily because, as always, he appeared to be coping so well.

When he suggested, unexpectedly, that we should perhaps put the parachute anchor in one evening, I was surprised. It was the first time he'd ever asked for that. Normally he would argue against it. The weather, although deteriorating, wasn't that bad yet. It was forecast to worsen, though, and night was closing in. There was little doubt we had another tough night ahead. Still, Sparky's suggestion we retreat onto the para anchor seemed out of character. I suspected there might be a problem.

'Are you OK, mate?' I asked. 'It's not like you to suggest putting the para anchor in early.'

He was a little defensive and, when I started to explain we needed to grab every mile possible, he finally told me what was bothering him.

'Mate, rowing at night in seas like the ones that smashed my oars is the most frightening thing I've ever done in my life. I'm not sure I can face much more of that.'

When a man who once picked up a guy in a minefield who'd had his leg blown off and then carried him to safety tells you he's never been as frightened in his life before, you tend to listen. When you're responsible for the thing that's scaring him, it also has a massive impact.

'Why didn't you say something, mate? I had no idea you were having any problems.'

'I didn't want to wimp out, mate, but after that knock down, rowing at night in big seas is scaring the shit out of me. I just can't see the big stuff coming and I'm spending the whole time worrying that I'm going to get smashed again like the last time.'

I was angry with myself. I couldn't believe I hadn't picked up on this. I felt sick to the stomach that I'd let him down again. Working with Sparky and watching him operate on the boat so effectively, I'd once more fallen into the trap of taking his capabilities for granted. I'd begun to think that, despite his condition, he could cope with anything that came along. Sparky's greatest qualities, his relentless positivity and can-do attitude, were proving to be at times his Achilles' heel. It was all too easy to assume he was indestructible.

What compounded the problem was that we hadn't had just the one bad night when the boat was knocked down, or even two. They had become so regular they were almost the norm. There'd been numerous nights equally as challenging and it seemed there was no end to them. The cumulative effect mentally on Sparky, knowing that at any moment the next monster wave could catch him out, must have been increasingly terrifying.

We had become a little more cautious, if only to protect the last remaining set of oars. But my natural competitive streak, which Sparky more than shared, had still encouraged us to push for as much distance as we could whenever possible. I should have known better.

He told me a story one night, as we rode out yet another a gale on the para anchor, which completely summed up not only his remarkably positive approach to his loss of vision but at the same time the soul destroying and at times heart-breaking reality of it.

After Blind Veterans had finally repatriated Sparky to the UK and his rehabilitation training had begun, he was offered the chance to study for a degree in physiotherapy. A natural athlete and a gifted sportsman, it was an obvious fit. He passed the entry exam, as ever, with flying colours and subsequently relocated to a university in London that, in conjunction with Blind Veterans, was pioneering the degree course.

'It was great, Mick, but it was just too soon. They really weren't ready for visually impaired people,' he said.

He explained that there was mountains of literature, with no practical way for a visually impaired person to easily study it. Even the equipment they were using for treatment wasn't designed for visually impaired people to use easily.

At one stage of the course there was an exam where the students had to demonstrate different muscle groups on the human body and the muscles' jobs. This was done by attaching electrodes to a volunteer and stimulating the muscle groups with a small electrical charge. This took place in a large medical theatre with all the other students looking on from the surrounding seats.

Sparky had been asked to isolate and activate the muscles which cause a person's arm to raise.

A friend of his had volunteered to be his patient and was laid on a trolley in the middle of the theatre with his shirt off. Sparky attached the various electrodes to him in the appropriate places and turned to the machine which controlled the electrical flow.

'The problem was, Mick, this machine was set up for a normally sighted person. There was nothing to help me to confirm what setting the electrical charge was on.'

I had a horrible feeling I knew where this story was going.

'Long story short,' he said, matter-of-factly, 'I activated the machine and, unfortunately, I'd put it on the highest setting, not the lowest. My mate's arm shot up like a rocket and hit me in the chest, sending me flying across the room, knocking a trolley over and leaving me on my arse covered in medical equipment. Meanwhile my mate was in shock, apparently with his hair sticking up, clutching his chest. He thought I'd tried to electrocute him. They had to rush him to A & E to make sure I hadn't damaged his heart. The whole bloody place was in uproar, everybody laughing their tits off,' he said straight-faced. 'They just weren't set up for blind people to do the course that first year.'

I remember the tears literally rolling down my cheeks when he first told me that story on the row. Remarkably, though, the lasting memory I have from hearing it has nothing to do with the events he described. A few moments after he'd finished recounting the story, when I'd finally stopped laughing, Sparky added, suddenly quite reflective, 'The thing is, Mick, things like that, as funny as they are, they start to shatter your confidence after a while.'

That last sentence felt like a kick in the stomach. I realised, perhaps for the first time, the frustrating reality of coping with sight loss. By its very nature a daily battle not to be confined by the condition, not to give in to it and withdraw from life, not to stop taking chances simply because the risk of failure was that much greater. If Sparky's confidence could be shaken by those inevitable setbacks, how must it be for people who didn't possess his almost superhuman levels of positivity?

The potential significance of our row and what it could mean for other people struggling with their own issues, not just visual impairment, began to sink in even more. If Sparky stepped off *Bo* in Honolulu as the first visually impaired person to have successfully rowed the Pacific, he would become a shining example for taking life by the scruff of the neck and striving to achieve your goals despite any perceived disability.

Sparky's achievement would put the daily challenges of anyone coming to terms with sight loss into perspective. It would promote an 'if Sparky can row the Pacific, I can bloody well get out and learn to use a bus' mentality. If we failed, however, it could easily reinforce the opposite reaction, that failure and limitations were the natural bedfellows to disability.

There was no middle ground. We had to be successful. It was an enormous added pressure which I'd never felt on any of my previous rows. Failure simply wasn't an option for Sparky and me.

Now fully aware of Sparky's understandable concern rowing in big seas at night, I adjusted our routine. It was a simple fix and it wouldn't have much of an impact on our progress. The next problem would, though.

It was approaching 10 p.m. on 15 July. The weather had improved, with lighter winds and calmer seas, although, as ever, it was still grey and overcast. Sparky had finished his stint on the oars. Once we'd swapped places and I was in place at the rowing position, he sat down in the cockpit near the cabin hatch. I thought he just wanted to chat for a few minutes before he went in to sleep as we often did.

'Mick,' he said, 'I'm running short of tablets.'

'What tablets?'

'The ones I'm taking to keep my colitis in check. Steroids.'

With the worry concerning his heart scare just before the row and the measures we'd had to put in place on board to cope with any possible heart problem, I'd almost forgotten about Sparky's colitis. He'd mentioned it during the build-up but assured me it wasn't a major issue and that it was easily controllable with medication. I know now that Sparky hadn't wanted to make too much of a fuss about it in case it became a reason for the race organisers to prevent him going.

'How many tablets have you got left?' I asked.

'Thirty days' worth.'

We weren't even halfway to Hawaii yet and we'd been at sea for thirty-nine days. My heart sank. There was every chance once we reached the elusive easterly trade winds our pace would increase, despite our shorter oars, but thirty days was still an optimistic target.

'How serious a problem is your colitis?' I asked, alarmed.

'Well. I've nearly died from it twice,' he answered evenly.

I nearly fell off the rowing seat. 'What? I had no idea it was that serious.'

'It's OK. Even if I run out of tablets, it doesn't mean I'll get a flare up straight away. I could be fine. It's been a couple of years since I've had any problems with it at all,' he said reassuringly.

'Right. So, what causes a flare up, then?' I asked, a little relieved.
'Stress.'

I fell forwards across the oars in front of me, laughing ironically. The alternative was to cry. 'Stress! Oh, we'll be fine, then, because it's not very stressful out here, is it?'

There was a pause. 'So, do you reckon we'll make it in inside thirty days?'

I smiled, shaking my head. 'It's possible but, if I'm honest, doubtful.' I thought some more.

'Look,' I said, 'as it stands, nothing's changed. If we make good time it won't even become an issue. If things change in the next few days, if we're behind schedule, we'll find a solution then.'

He seemed happy with that. It seemed like a sensible plan.

At midnight, Sparky emerged from the cabin for our changeover. We swapped positions and I prepared to get some sleep. Before I disappeared into the cabin, Sparky said ominously, 'There's another problem, Mick.'

I braced myself for bad news.

'My knee is totally knackered. I can't row.'

I'd spent the whole of my last two-hour watch working out the time permutations of reaching Hawaii before the precious supply of steroids controlling Sparky's colitis was exhausted, eventually convincing myself that, with a bit of luck, we could reach the finish line before the drugs ran out. There was, it had seemed, light at the end of an increasingly dark tunnel. In one sentence that light had now been extinguished.

'What do you mean you can't row?' I asked. 'What's the problem?'

'Every time I pull myself back on the rowing seat when my leg extends, it's agony.' Apparently, he'd been battling with the increasingly painful problem for some time.

'What about some painkillers?' I suggested.

'I'm not taking painkillers. That'll just mask the problem and make it worse,' he fired back sharply. Sparky eventually admitted to me he was more concerned a course of painkillers might aggravate his colitis.

'Mate,' I said, 'on an ocean rowing boat, painkillers are only ever going to mask the problem. There's not much that's actually going to get better out here. We just need to mask the problem until we get to dry land.'

He was unconvinced, but eventually agreed to take some ibuprofen, the same tablets I'd taken for my shoulder injury, to see if it helped. He needed to rest because he was in too much pain to row. More worryingly, he didn't seem himself. He wasn't making a lot of sense when I was talking to him and he appeared utterly exhausted. I thought sleep deprivation might be a big part of the problem.

With the clock ticking at thirty days to get in, and now the possibility of half the rowing output disappearing, there was little chance I was going to sleep during my two hours off. I told him to get some more sleep in the cabin while I carried on rowing and worked out a plan. That night I chose the phrase 'death of a thousand cuts' to describe our voyage.

At ten o'clock the next day, after one of the toughest nights I'd experienced on a rowing boat, things were beginning to look up. The rest had done Sparky good and the painkillers had worked. The pain in his knee had subsided and he was more his normal self. There was one more problem, though.

The index finger on his right hand was badly swollen, with what appeared to be an infected cut on the knuckle.

'How does that look, Mick?' he asked.

'Well, it's put me off my breakfast,' I answered. 'We need to clean that up and get some antibiotics in you immediately, mate.'

His finger was a mess, swollen and red, with puss oozing out of the wound.

The cut wasn't particularly serious, just a knock where he'd broken the skin. The infection which had set in, though, was very serious, particularly in the conditions we were living in. I didn't say anything to Sparky at the time, but I was far more concerned about his finger than I was about his knee.

At worst his knee injury would simply prevent him rowing if it deteriorated. If the infection in his finger wasn't dealt with, it could have far more serious implications. I rifled through the medical kit looking for suitable antibiotics. Ciprofloxacin seemed to fit the bill. We started the course of antibiotics immediately and cleaned the wound and dressed it.

With Sparky's various ailments and injuries hopefully now under control, we returned to our relentless rowing routine once more in order to drag ourselves as swiftly as possible to Hawaii.

The next few days brought painfully slow progress. Lighter winds set in and the temperature increased at least during the day, but annoyingly it was still bitterly cold at night. Frustratingly, we could feel the lack of power in each stroke we took with the shorter oars. It was like driving a car in third gear. I estimated we were probably losing 20 or 30 per cent of our potential daily mileage, while expending the same amount of energy. That constant realisation and the relentlessly exhausting rowing routine made for a subdued atmosphere on board.

On the positive side, Sparky's knee was holding up. It was far from 100 per cent, but he could at least row, albeit a more restricted stroke. More importantly, the infection in his knuckle seemed to be responding well to the antibiotics. On the downside, I was becoming increasingly aware the possibility of us reaching Hawaii before his steroid tablets ran out was unlikely.

I asked tentatively, 'How many of those steroid tablets do you take each day, Sparky?'

'Four,' he answered.

'Right, how about we reduce that to three a day? Would that be possible? That would give us another week or more to play with. If you feel any reaction, we could always up the dose again straight away.'

'We could try it,' he answered cautiously.

If at any point Sparky had developed symptoms of colitis, I'd have immediately initiated an emergency recovery. For now, though, both of us agreed we would do all we could to keep the row on track. We'd keep on finding a way, until there were no other options left. Worryingly, though, those options seemed to be disappearing.

We were almost at the halfway mark, at least in terms of distance. I was also approaching my five hundredth day at sea in an ocean rowing boat. There are only a handful of people in the world who are members of that unique ocean rowing club. In all that time at sea I'd never once felt the pressure I was feeling now rowing in the Great Pacific Race with Sparky. I felt myself crumbling beneath the weight of the responsibility and the seemingly endless setbacks we were having to deal with. I'd been concerned at the beginning of the project I might have bitten off more than I could chew financially. I'd battled through that and got to the start line by the skin of my teeth. Now en route to Hawaii, for the first time in my life I began to consider that I may have bitten off more than I could chew rowing.

CHAPTER 26

PAIN AND ISOLATION

At some point during 20 July, after forty-five days at sea, we passed the halfway mark in terms of distance between Monterey Bay and Honolulu geographically. It had little significance for me. I didn't even note the hour in the log. It would, after all, only serve as the halfway point once we'd successfully finished the row. That was by no means a foregone conclusion yet. Increasingly, it seemed, far from it.

The weather had continued to be depressingly overcast, and although the winds were lighter, their direction was no more helpful. To make matters worse, I discovered two spare cannisters of gas for our cooker appeared to have been left behind in California. We'd been heating up every one of our meals, including the desserts, throughout the voyage due to the temperatures we'd been experiencing. Suddenly, with the extended time at sea to look forward to and the unexpected loss of two spare canisters, we were running short of fuel for the cooking.

'Right, no more hot desserts, mate,' I informed Sparky. Worse than that, though, we also had to reduce the amount of tea we were drinking. This was particularly frustrating as a friend had provided us with 1600 teabags for the voyage, just so we didn't run out. One positive: our food package was made up of Expedition Foods products, specifically designed dehydrated food ideal for ocean rows. The meals were varied, tasty and calorific, and they were also easily rehydrated with cold water. It just took a little longer. We could still eat no matter what.

'I can cope without hot food,' Sparky said. 'But not without a hot wet of tea.' He was a man after my own heart!

The rowing regime continued to be brutal. There was nothing but long hard days and nights at the oars with painfully little in terms of mileage to show for it. The only upside was Sparky's knee seemed to be holding up and the infection in the wound to his finger was responding to the antibiotics. Even more importantly, there was no adverse reaction to the reduction in steroid tablets Sparky was taking each day.

We were both constantly exhausted, though, and it eventually began to tell on us. I emerged from the cabin early one morning to relieve Sparky, and I realised immediately things weren't quite as they should be. He was sitting at the rowing position moving forwards and backwards on the rowing seat, but neither blade was actually entering the water during his stroke. I wondered absentmindedly how long he might have been rowing like this for.

'I've been caught by a current,' Sparky said animatedly, when he heard me emerge on deck.

'It's dragged me into this village,' he said, as if that would explain why we were in a village in the middle of the Pacific Ocean. 'We're miles off course, mate. A camper van has just gone past me.'

'Mate, I think you need some sleep. There aren't any villages around here and definitely no camper vans,' I said, smiling, thinking back to what Riggs had had to put up with from me on the Yukon when I'd started hallucinating.

'Do you not think those oars would work better if you put them in the water at some point?' I added, chuckling.

He didn't even register my comment. 'We're miles off course, mate,' he insisted. 'This current's taken us miles out of the way!'

I encouraged him off the rowing seat and got him back into the cabin. He needed to get some sleep and a proper rest. I rowed through the morning until lunch just to give him time to fully recover. He emerged later in the day largely oblivious to what had happened at the changeover but very much himself again.

'Wake me in a couple of hours,' I said, before crawling into the cabin.

Sparky rowed the whole of the afternoon without waking me. I must have been exhausted – I slept for over four hours before realising I was late for my watch.

'Mate, you should have shouted me,' I said, angry with myself for sleeping through the changeover.

'It's a team effort, mate. You let me get some sleep, I'm repaying the favour.'

I grinned knowingly. It was the definition of the principle which got Chris Martin and me across the North Pacific: each of us putting the other first. It's the basic foundation on which great teams are built. If you work with someone who continually demonstrates they're putting you first, it's contagious. You want to do the same for them. That creates a positive upward spiral that inevitably builds a team which is greater than the sum of its parts. Chris and I were definitely far greater than the sum of our parts on the North Pacific. We had to be. I was pleased to see it was working again for Sparky and me.

It's a principle that organisations like the Royal Marines rely on, and it's one of the first lessons taught when you join you up. 'Put your oppo first.' It protects the group, makes the individual and the team stronger, and it works. I had no doubt Sparky would have that quality engrained in his character when we came up with the idea of rowing the Pacific. I suspect he had that quality even before he joined up. It was one of the reasons I was so confident we'd be successful. It was still gratifying to see it so ably demonstrated, though. It was a principle which we'd lean heavily on during the remainder of the voyage.

The day after Sparky's amusing hallucinations I checked our position prior to my watch, around midnight. It showed we'd headed north several miles during the previous two hours. It made no sense and didn't tally with the wind, the direction the boat was facing or the course Sparky was rowing.

I thought maybe Sparky had rowed off course, but in fact he hadn't. We'd entered a northly flow of water and it had taken us with it. Sparky had been rowing in one direction but the current had taken us in another. After weeks of being pushed too far south and finally reaching some easterly winds, we were now charting a course directly towards the Hawaiian Islands. Too much north in our course now and we could easily miss them. We needed to put a little south into our course once again as we travelled west.

I could already imagine the headlines in the newspapers: 'Blind man rowing the Pacific misses Hawaii'. It didn't bear thinking about.

To my relief, it proved to be an isolated and narrow strip of current. We eventually managed to cross it without losing too many more miles north and resumed our course to Honolulu. It was one more added pressure, though, to add to the countless others.

It was 27 July, the day we passed the last 1000 miles mark. It was positive news, but I knew better than anyone that 1000 miles in an ocean rowing boat is plenty of time for things to go wrong.

I was sleeping in the cabin late in the afternoon when I heard a terrible scream outside. It was Sparky, obviously in severe pain. As

I emerged hurriedly from the cabin, I saw he was bent double over the oars and for a split second I thought that he was having a heart attack.

'My back,' he cried in a strangled voice. 'I've snapped something in my back.' He was obviously in a lot of pain. I moved out on deck to help him, securing the oars and trying to make him comfortable. He was crippled. He could barely move.

'My back,' he said again breathlessly. 'It sounded like a shot going off. Somethings snapped across my shoulders'

He leaned forwards and I checked his back. I found nothing at first, then running my hand lower down his shoulder I discovered a lump the size of a billiard ball under the skin, about halfway between his spine and his shoulder joint.

'Arrrr!' He grimaced. 'That's it. What the fuck have I done now?'

We contacted the race HQ to let them know what had happened and get some advice. Eventually a diagnosis of a likely compression fracture was suggested by their excellent on-call doctor Aeynor Sawyer. Tissue had snapped, bringing with it a part of the bone.

It seemed his efforts to compensate for his injured knee while he'd been rowing had caused an unnatural strain on part of his back and ultimately resulted in this very painful, debilitating injury. Fortunately, although in great pain, he wasn't in any immediate danger or risk of further injury.

With almost a thousand miles to go to the finish line, our rowing capacity had just been cut in half. 'He needs painkillers and rest,' Aeynor advised. 'He may be able to row again before you reach Hawaii but I suspect it's unlikely, Mick. It will certainly be a couple of weeks before he's even able to think about that.'

She asked me to send through an update on his condition together with his vital signs every four hours, just to be on the safe side.

He was already on painkillers. The only alternative if they didn't help was to move him on to more powerful drugs. Tramadol, a narcotic, would be the next step up.

'Let's see how he goes for now with what he's taking,' Aeynor suggested. 'We can look at that later if we need to.'

Despite his injury, Sparky was still remarkably positive. He didn't want to get off the boat, which would have been most people's first reaction. He understood the nature of the injury and was confident that he could eventually get back on the oars before we arrived. We set up a new solo rowing routine, where I would row for a minimum of four hours and then rest for up to three. Our race was now purely an exercise in getting to Honolulu.

Sparky insisted, despite his injury, that on my off time he'd vacate the cabin so I could get some proper sleep without us both being crammed inside together. It would prove to be an enormous help – the weather was becoming warmer and the cabin a claustrophobic sweatbox when we both were in there together.

After I finished my first longer stint on the oars, I retreated to the cabin for a much-needed rest. The mileage was limited when I was rowing with our underpowered oars. We barely moved at all when I wasn't rowing, despite the wind increasingly blowing from the east.

It was soul destroying. The reality of yet another setback to overcome was almost overwhelming. One after another, each of these seemingly endless problems was adding on days to our projected finish date. It felt almost like we were going backwards.

Sparky's injury would likely mean it would now take us close to three months to complete a row which originally we'd been aiming to finish in fifty-six days or less. I was beginning to feel utterly crushed by the pressure to reach this increasingly elusive finish line.

In 2004, attempting to row solo across the North Pacific from Japan, I found myself trapped in my sinking boat after I was capsized over a thousand miles away from San Francisco. Despite the potentially lethal circumstances I was in, I steadfastly refused to pray for help to get out of the situation. I believed that, if I was meant to survive, I would have the ability to do so without asking some faceless deity to help me. I didn't want to be one of those people who suddenly gets religion when he thinks it'll save his skin.

I'm not proud to admit that, for the first time ever, I prayed for help in that cabin less than a thousand miles from Hawaii. My only excuse is I wasn't asking for help for myself, I was asking for help getting Sparky to the finish line. I wanted to make good on my promise to get us to Honolulu, and I was beginning to believe I wasn't capable of making that happen. For the first time ever on an ocean rowing boat, even a sinking one, I thought I might be beat. An old family friend Ted Eglin, a veteran of D-Day, had once said to me, 'Everybody prays in the end, Mick.' It seemed he was right, because I did. I prayed for help.

Make of this what you will, but only hours later we found ourselves in a powerful ocean current taking us due west towards Hawaii. Despite being down to one rower we were making greater speed towards the islands than at any other time on the voyage. I'm not sure if it was a miracle, but it bloody well felt like one. There was a part of me that suspected if I'd looked up at the sky at that moment there'd have been a white-bearded figure grinning down at me saying, 'Gotcha!'

Regardless, that turn of events, divine or otherwise, pulled me back from the brink of defeat and brought Hawaii within our grasp once more. I'm not sure if I was any more religious after that experience, but I was very grateful.

My five hundredth day on an ocean rowing boat came on 3 August. This would have been my dad's birthday if he'd still been alive. Dave Bull, one of our stalwart supporters back at The Coach House in Rottingdean had given us a small flask of port to toast the key points of the voyage. Sparky and I each raised a small tumbler to my dad and my ocean rowing milestone.

'Hopefully we're not going to be out here for your six hundredth day,' Sparky said sarcastically.

We'd managed to remain in the miraculously helpful current for several days, even negotiating a perilous change of direction it made, jinking slightly further south, without losing it. The helpful extra mileage it afforded us compensated for Sparky's injury, but it was still very tough going. For Sparky particularly so.

For me the rowing routine was actually easier than the two hours on, two off had been. On top of the rowing, the cooking and navigating and any extra jobs had to be done around that rota, eating into my two hours off. Although rowing more hours now, it was not at the same intensity and I was actually getting more sleep.

Perversely, for Sparky, still in considerable pain from his back injury and unable to row at all, life was becoming almost unbearable. He was basically locked in the cabin while I was rowing, or sitting alone on the deck when I was sleeping. Without the routine and rigorous demands of the rowing, life on board was becoming mind-numbingly boring for him, to the point of mental torture.

To try to fend off boredom caused by Sparky not being able to see birds and fish and waves as mental stimulation, we had brought along musical playlists.

Our playlist had been created by Nat's dad, Mr H. We had given him an outline of the kind of music we both liked – broadly speaking, 'old music' – and he promptly put together an eclectic and lengthy playlist of tracks and albums based on that. We both loved it. There was one awkward moment, however, when we were on deck with the music playing in the background and Sparky suddenly asked, 'Do you and Nat's dad get on, Mick?'

I was taken aback by the question. 'Yes, I think so,' I answered.

'He's OK about you and her becoming an item, then?' he said questioningly.

'I think so,' I replied. 'Why?'

'Well. If I'm not mistaken, this is the theme tune from *Titanic*. I thought he might be trying to tell you something,' he replied, laughing.

That minor glitch apart, the playlist had been a success, at least it had when we'd both been rowing. The problem was Sparky needed a far greater variety of entertainment and stimulation now he wasn't able to row. We simply didn't have it.

I made a throwaway comment to him one day, joking about it being all right for him, loafing in the cabin all day while I was doing all the work. He nearly jumped down my throat, his frustration and boredom suddenly coming to the fore.

'You've no idea what it's like for me stuck in here all day every day,' he shouted angrily. 'It's like being in a fucking pitch-black cell in solitary confinement. I'm going out of my head. I'd give anything to be rowing.'

Once again, I hadn't appreciated what Sparky was having to deal with. The boredom and increasing isolation were compounded by the constant pain from his back injury. He also had the worry that at any time he might suffer an attack of colitis. He had an awful lot on his plate.

'Mate,' I said, not for the first time, 'why didn't you tell me? You don't need to be locked in there. Open that hatch and speak to me. I'm only out here and happy to chat whenever you want.'

Yet again I'd been oblivious to the unique problems Sparky faced as a direct result of his vision impairment. Now I made a conscious decision to start chatting to Sparky more often and describe in detail what was going on around the boat. It wasn't long before I got my first opportunity.

By this stage we'd picked up a school of dorado which were living beneath *Bo*. These are strikingly beautiful fish with a blue-green colour. They can grow up to two metres in length, although our visitors seemed only about half that size. They must have numbered over a hundred, the most I've ever seen together. They were a colourful and spectacular sight around the boat. Descending deep beneath the ocean during the day, at night they came to the surface to feed on the large numbers of flying fish which now seemed to surround our boat. Being hit in the head by a flying fish trying to avoid an unpleasant fate at the hands of the dorado was becoming an occupational hazard of rowing. We were also seemingly a focal point for bird life. There was an unusually wide variety of different species of birds making the most of the abundance of flying fish.

On one occasion, shortly after Sparky told me about how tough it was dealing with the boredom, we were both sitting on deck. I was cooking a meal. He was opposite near the cabin hatch, facing towards me. Over his shoulder I watched a large flying fish, maybe eight- or ten-inches long, launch into the air from the water, presumably in an effort to avoid one of the dorado. As it took flight, a bird swooped down to grab it. Amazingly, the fish changed direction at the last moment and managed to avoid the attack. I was watching a bizarre kind of aerial dogfight, with the fish skilfully or luckily avoiding the bird's repeated attempts to get it in its clutches. This remarkable spectacle went on for several more seconds before, victorious, the fish disappeared unscathed beneath the surface of the ocean. I described it as best I could to Sparky as the action unfolded behind him.

In more than five hundred days at sea I'd never seen anything like it before. This, to me, is the appeal of ocean rowing – on any given day you may see something unique and quite incredible.

Sparky's shoulder was still proving painful. An ocean rowing boat isn't the best place to recover from any injury, least of all one which can be aggravated by any sudden movement. Ocean rowing boats are constantly moving. The pain was darkening his mood and his inability to row was frustrating him. We spoke to Aeynor and she recommended taking the much stronger painkiller, Tramadol, so he could at least gain some respite from the discomfort.

Chris Martin, the race director, offered to send the support boat to rescue us if we wished.

'I'm pretty certain I know what your answer's going to be,' he said, 'but I thought I'd ask.'

'Yeah.' I laughed. 'We've already discussed this option, mate. We'll pass on that for now if it's all the same to you,' I replied politely. 'It's bad, but it's not that bad.'

After over two months at sea, I noted in the log on 8 August that I rowed at night for the first time without wearing my waterproof jacket. By then we'd even begun to experience a few hot sunny days.

Only a week or so after Sparky's injury I noticed something odd. Every time I emerged from the cabin to row again, the oars which I'd pulled in and stowed across the boat at the rowing position seemed to have been resecured. Somebody had untied them and presumably put them back in the water again. Sparky was obviously trying to see if he was able to row. It was remarkable, as at that stage he was struggling just to get in and out of the cabin.

'How's the rowing going?' I asked out of the blue one morning.

He looked up shocked. 'How do you know I've been trying to row?' he asked, surprised.

'Your knots are shit, mate. I can see when you've retied the line securing the blades,' I replied, laughing.

He shrugged. 'I'm still fucked, Mick. I can't put any real pressure into the stroke,' he said despondently. 'But I'll keep trying.'

'That's hardly surprising.' I laughed. 'It's barely a week since you had the injury, mate. Don't mess yourself up trying to get back on the oars too soon. All you've got to be fit for is to row us across the finish line off Honolulu and into the Waikiki Yacht Club. Anything else is a bonus,' I said encouragingly.

'I'll do better than that, Mick, I can promise you that,' he replied earnestly.

Our progress was still steady. We'd managed to remain in the current which we had been miraculously provided with at just the right time. Its speed was decreasing as we closed on the islands, though, and I knew it would soon weaken and die. Sparky was now taking Tramadol most days to reduce the pain in his shoulder. The pain was less but he was increasingly withdrawn. We were still on course to make the finish line, but there was no question we would be much later than anticipated.

By 11 August the current which had brought us such relief finally disappeared and died away. Our daily mileage decreased depressingly with its departure. With still over 400 miles to go, it made for a sombre mood on board once again.

Sparky was still unable to row, but he'd insisted on helping with other jobs on board. He'd pumped out all the deck lockers, which had invariably taken on water, and he serviced both sets of wheels on the two rowing seats we had on board. The in-line skate wheels we used on the seats were beginning to break down with constant use. Both jobs were a massive help for me as they were time consuming and energy sapping. I had noticed, though, that Sparky seemed to have slipped back into a quiet and withdrawn mood again. He wasn't talking much and I was becoming concerned. A day or so later a stupid argument blew up out of nothing. I think it was something as trivial as getting in each other's way changing positions on the deck. Whatever it was, it served as a flash point.

It was simply a release valve for the pressure we were both increasingly feeling by that time. With Hawaii and the finish now approaching, the financial pressures which the project still had hanging over it were starting to dominate my thoughts. There were a number of bills yet to pay and little money left in the sponsorship pot. I would need to deal with the reality of that very soon.

Sparky, on the other hand, simply wanted to be able to row again and help get us over the finish line as quickly as possible. It was only a matter of time before this had to come to a head. The argument was over as quickly as it begun, raised voices and few heated words, none of which applied to any of the problems either of us were actually dealing with. Sparky retired silently to the cabin. I returned to my rowing.

Nikki, Sparky's partner, had laughingly told me before we left that her only concern about the trip was, 'When me and Sparky have a row, he likes to go for a walk on his own to get over it. Then he's right as rain. There's nowhere to go for a walk on a rowing boat, Mick.'

She was right. The atmosphere on board became unbearably tense after the fall out. Sparky didn't have anywhere to go for a walk, and he certainly didn't want to talk to me. We spent the next twenty-four hours in almost total silence. I realised I had to try to do something to defuse the situation before it blew up out of all proportion.

At the next changeover I bit the bullet and apologised to Sparky.

'If I've been out of order or said something that's offended you, mate, I'm sorry,' I said.

I made it clear to him there were few people who had more respect for him than me before we started the row, and none had more respect now. I wasn't lying. It had been a humbling and inspirational experience watching Sparky deal with the seemingly endless problems we'd faced. Not many normally sighted people could have coped.

'We've come through everything that's been thrown at us and we're just days away from finishing. Let's not fuck that all up with a pointless argument now, mate,' I said.

He nodded and acknowledged what I said, but didn't respond.

'One other thing, mate,' I said, 'and don't take this the wrong way. You might want to think about not taking Tramadol for a few days. I know it's stopping the pain, but I don't think it's doing you any favours mentally.'

The following morning, I'm pleased to say, it was if the argument had never happened. Sparky had taken my advice and skipped the next dose of Tramadol, replacing it with ibuprofen. I don't know if this was the reason, but his mood was brighter. He was happier, chatting again and back on form. He was even talking about getting back on the oars for an hour or two here and there to see how he got on.

I breathed a huge sigh of relief. The voyage had thrown up enough challenges along the way, and we didn't need to be adding to them with problems of our own making. We were little more than a week away from finishing, if we were lucky. We should be enjoying these last few days of what had become a remarkable voyage. What neither of us could know then was that we were about to face our biggest challenge yet, a potentially project-ending and life-threatening one.

Hurricane Lane was about to show up.

CHAPTER 27

BATTLING LANE

We had almost two days before the brunt force of Hurricane Lane was likely to reach us. I believed this would be ample time to prepare. In some ways, it was too much time. Although confident we could survive what was coming, the responsibility of another person's life hanging in the balance weighed heavily on me.

Every hour that passed dragged terribly. I constantly asked myself, Have I made the right decision? I was confident I had, but an element of doubt is the natural bedfellow to any life-or-death decision. Our window for rescue had passed. It was too late to change our minds. There was no getting off now.

Sparky and I used the time well, setting up the boat as best as we could to deal with the approaching storm. She was designed to cope with the rigors of the Pacific, and she had already done so for over two long, arduous months, so I knew we couldn't have been aboard a better ocean rowing boat for the job.

Sparky filled up two of the central lockers, which had once contained our rations, with salt water. This replaced the lost ballast of the consumed food and created additional ballast, so we sat lower and more solidly in the water. With our parachute anchor deployed from the stern of the boat, we would also sit with the stern facing into the ferocious waves and winds the hurricane delivered, and we would be far less susceptible to capsize. It would be a scary and violently uncomfortable experience, but likely a survivable one. I hoped.

As the hours ticked by, the oppressive grey clouds heralding Lane's approach began to dominate the vast sky above the ocean.

The windspeed steadily increased, and squalls of heavy rain show-ers regularly swept over us. Bizarrely, considering the first five weeks of the voyage had been notable for the bitter cold, it was now uncomfortably hot. Crammed into the cabin together as we sheltered from the increasingly dangerous weather, the climate was almost unbearable.

With the prospect of at least another twenty-four hours locked in the cabin as the peak of the storm roared over us, I decided to go out on deck to give us both a break from the claustrophobic conditions inside. I unfastened the hatch.

As I stepped into the cockpit and closed the hatch behind me, I nearly had a heart attack! There was a huge ship no more than a couple of hundred metres away, crashing through the ocean, its bow leaping forty, fifty feet into the air as it ploughed directly through the oncoming waves. It was far too close to our tiny craft for comfort. Although it didn't look immediately like it was on a direct collision course, I had to make sure. If it came close enough, its bow wave could roll us, and closer than that would mean impact, either of which could prove fatal. I scrambled back into the compartment and grabbed the VHF radio, trying to explain to Sparky as I did so.

Luckily, I was able to hail the unidentified ship. Much to my relief, the officer on watch responded almost immediately and confirmed he'd seen our position on his radar, thanks to our AIS (automatic identifying system) transmitter. In the worsening conditions, he had only just managed to locate us visually as we disappeared in and out of the growing swell and the roaring waves.

He informed me that every port in the Hawaiian Islands had now closed, with all the ships previously docked there rousted to sea to avoid encountering the coming storm. He was only one of many huge commercial vessels now making their way north and east away from the destructive path of Lane. Many of those ships would be steaming directly past our position, making the risk of collision a major concern as the storm steadily grew.

'The next twenty-four hours are going to be very tough for you, but if you get through that, it should steadily begin to improve,' he informed me unemotionally, one mariner to another. We were both aware of the constant battle waged against our common adversary, the ocean, and the risks inherent with so powerful a force.

I wished my faceless friend good luck and replaced the handset. I took a last look at the crashing waves growing all around us and realised Lane had officially arrived. I slipped back into the unappealing cabin that was our only refuge and wondered what the next day would bring.

We'd been stranded on the parachute anchor for almost three days, riding out the steadily increasing winds and seas, before Lane finally hit. We were 164 miles from the finish line, and before we deployed the anchor, due to the trade winds and accompanying bands of helpful current, making our best daily mileage of the race. We greeted Lane's arrival with equal measures of trepidation and relief.

Sparky was still in a lot of pain from his shoulder injury and, to add more worry, he only had one more day of steroid tablets left to stave off an attack or colitis. Whatever happened now he was going to be spending several more days at sea with nothing to prevent a potentially lethal attack of his illness setting in.

'Normally it takes time to develop if I have an attack. It doesn't just come on in hours. It'll take days,' he assured me.

I hoped there'd be at least four of those days, as that was how long it would likely take us to reach the finish line once Lane passed.

The close proximity of the finish line was, frustratingly, all the more obvious by virtue of the fact I could see land. The Big Island had come into view a day or two before we were forced onto the parachute anchor. The sighting was made easier courtesy of the clouds created by its currently erupting active volcano. Dave Bull, who'd provided our small supply of port, had specifically requested we toast the moment when we both saw land again.

'Woohoo!' I'd shouted when I realised what I was seeing in the very far distance between the clouds. 'I've seen land, I can see the Big Island's volcano. Get out the port!'

'Dave said when we both see land,' Sparky said flatly. 'I can't see anything yet.'

'Well, I suppose you've got a point there,' I replied deflated.

It would be several days yet before Sparky would sight land with his severely limited vision. Those days would see a host of other adventures before we could finally raise those two hard-earned tumblers of port in a toast to the Hawaiian Islands.

We weren't the only ones braving the advancing hurricane in the days leading up to Lane's arrival. Nat and Nikki found themselves on an unsurprisingly sparsely populated connecting flight from Los Angeles to Hawaii. The islands were moving towards full lockdown and it would only be a matter of time before the airports closed completely. As we rode out the early effects of Lane's approach on board *Bo*, the girls passed high and directly above us, anxious to arrive safely on the island of Oahu before Lane rendered that impossible.

It was a scenario we thought highly unlikely until just a couple of weeks earlier. I knew Nat was intending to be at the finish, but the costs for Nikki to join her were prohibitive. The project budget, long since exhausted, had nothing left to help with the cost, and there was the very real prospect Sparky would step ashore having rowed the Pacific Ocean and not be able to share that incredible moment with Nikki.

The Royal Marines Charity were not about to let that happen, though. They contacted Nikki and said they would cover the cost of her flight. They recognised the incredible achievement Sparky was on the verge of completing and felt he should be able to celebrate that with Nikki, his partner. It was a remarkable and generous gesture, which for me summed up the family ethos that The Royal Marines Charity rightly champions. It was also a huge morale booster for Sparky when he heard the good news.

We were also informed there was a Royal Marine brigadier on secondment to the North Pacific Command with the American forces in Hawaii. His name was Rory Copinger-Symes. The Royal Marine Charity had been in touch with him and he was banging the drum on the island ahead of our anticipated arrival. He already had great news for us – the Ala Moana Hotel on Oahu had offered to sponsor our stay once we arrived. We no longer had to worry about finding or funding accommodation when we landed. It was one less pressure.

Despite the litany of setbacks on the row itself, and the ominous spectre of Lane lumbering towards us, it seemed finally our luck was changing for the better. Then completely unexpectedly news came which confirmed beyond all doubt our luck had indeed changed for the better, all because of Hurricane Lane.

Becca Saunders, who runs her own public relations agency, Unique PR and Marketing, contacted me by satellite phone. Becca is an old and long-suffering friend from my early ocean rowing days. She'd agreed to take on the public relations for the first Cockleshell Endeavour adventures with Steve Grenham. Four highly unprofitable years later, at least from her perspective, she'd still been unable to extricate herself from our adventures. The work she'd done for Sparky and me leading up to the race had been outstanding, giving us a national profile with articles and interviews on TV and radio across the UK prior to our departure. She was, though, about to exceed even her own high standards.

'Mick,' she said on the satellite phone, 'great news. The US media have got hold of the fact that a Brit blind veteran is rowing the Pacific and he's now in the path of the Cat 5 hurricane about to hit Hawaii. The response has been bonkers. I've got radio and national TV all over the States that want to speak to Sparky. I know you guys are busy, but could we arrange some phone interviews, please?'

It was the best news we could have had. It almost made the threat of Lane's imminent arrival bearable. Press coverage meant Sparky's exploits would reach a wider international audience. It was fantastic news.

Besides, we were no longer that busy on board. We'd already prepared *Bo* for the approaching storm. She was as ready as she'd ever be, as were we. Now it was simply a matter of waiting to discover what the hurricane had in store for us. Having the distraction of media attention and interviews would be a great way to kill time and a welcome morale booster for the pair of us.

In the twenty-four hours leading up to Lane's arrival, Sparky gave a wide range of interviews both to the US and UK media. He was a natural. His easy, self-depreciating, no-nonsense style made him an interviewer's dream. The process of talking about the row also seemed to finally bring home to Sparky the significance of what he was about to achieve.

I think by that stage we'd both become so worn down by the seemingly endless litany of setbacks we'd faced that we'd almost lost sight of the goal we were now so close to achieving. When Sparky stepped ashore in Waikiki as the first visually impaired person to row the Pacific Ocean, that would be a unique and remarkable achievement, something which could never be surpassed. There could only ever be one first blind man to row the Pacific Ocean. Sparky was on the verge of becoming that man.

Providing, of course, we survived the next twenty-four hours.

Lane eventually hit Oahu on the evening of the 24th. Luckily for us and the Hawaiian Islands, the hurricane's path changed slightly at the very last minute and the centre of the storm arched west just south of Oahu. That fortuitous change of direction enhanced our chances of survival immeasurably, and mercifully lessened the devastating impact all of the Hawaiian Islands had been bracing themselves for.

We'd battened down the hatches (yes, you actually do that in a severe storm) in what was the survivable quadrant of the storm. The drop in wind speeds as a result of that late change in Lane's direction, however slight, made that quadrant considerably *more* survivable. It was still a tough time on board *Bo* as the full effects of the storm finally hit, but a manageable one. From the afternoon of the 23rd through to early morning on the 24th, Sparky and I remained almost constantly locked in the cabin, squeezed together, constantly pummelled by the increasingly strong winds and seas Lane delivered.

Bizarrely, no matter how bad the weather becomes outside, the secure rear-cabin on an ocean rowing boat can seem like an oasis of calm. My brother and I had christened the cabin The Nest on our 2001 Atlantic crossing, because it always felt so secure, so detached from what was happening outside. Once securely in The Nest it was as if you had stepped into another world.

It was no different for Sparky and me almost two decades later. The cabin still felt like a deceptively secure cocoon distanced from the mounting chaos outside. The only difference was the temperature in the cabin meant it felt like we were living in a sauna.

We attempted to sleep through as much of the storm as we could, waking instantly whenever a particularly violent wave struck from an unexpected angle. *Bo*, as always, remained rock solid and seemingly invulnerable on the end of the parachute anchor. The stern of our trusty boat, to which the anchor was attached, facing resolutely into the ferocious winds and seas. Never once did she threaten to buckle or fail under the onslaught.

From time to time I eased the hatch open an inch or two to let some fresh air in and cool down the cabin's oppressively hot and humid atmosphere. We were immediately greeted by a terrifying increase in noise as Lane's voice, in all its roaring glory, could be heard.

Once you've spent even one moment in such a daunting environment, the mythical tales of beautiful sirens and their haunting voices tempting unsuspecting sailors to their doom make perfect sense. The powerful winds and waves combine to create a cacophony of terrifyingly melancholy wails. A terrified ancient mariner could easily be forgiven for rationalising such experiences with sinister and superstitious explanations. Mercifully, on board *Bo* we could achieve at least a partial separation from that terrifying world by simply closing the hatch.

CHAPTER 28

THE FINAL CUT

Mid-morning the next day I tentatively stepped out on deck for the first time since Lane's arrival. The sky was full of angry grey clouds and the wind was still blowing strongly, but it had lost its ferocity and the powerful gusts which had battered us during the night were gone.

Looking around the deck of *Bo*, everything seemed as it should, secure and still in place. The only obvious indicator of the night's dramas, our Union flag, or what was left of it, was now torn to shreds, twice as long as before but only three or four inches high. It had become a red, white and blue streamer tauntingly pointing directly towards our destination.

The night had been dreadful. It had been depressingly uncomfortable for me. I can only imagine how it must have been for Sparky with his injury. We were both at the point where we just wanted to get in and get off the boat.

I contacted Chris at the race HQ to let him know we'd come through the night unscathed and that we'd be retrieving the parachute anchor shortly and getting back on the oars.

He was relieved to hear from us and glad the night had gone well. He confirmed what we suspected. Lane's last-minute course diversion had reduced her impact on us and the islands. We weren't the only ones breathing a sigh of relief that morning. We and the whole of the Hawaiian Islands had dodged a bullet. It could have been much worse.

Chris confirmed that the weather forecast was still strong winds and rough seas, but with steadily improving conditions over the next few days. The worst had definitely passed. He added with a note of caution, 'The sea state in the channel between Molokai and Oahu is going to be very confused with a large chop when you get there. You'll need to be careful.'

The sea depth falls off from over 2000 metres to less than 450 in under 10 miles on the approach to the channel between the two islands. The huge seas generated by Lane would have funnelled directly along this stretch of water for several days now, creating a potentially very dangerous sea state. I made a mental note. That was still more than a hundred miles away, perhaps another three days rowing. Things would hopefully improve by then. With the passing of the hurricane, everybody including us began to think it was now a forgone conclusion we would reach the finish line and row into Waikiki Yacht Club.

Yet again we would discover the Pacific had other ideas.

Although the winds were now manageable and the sea had lost some of its ferocity, the conditions were still testing as we retrieved the parachute anchor for what we hoped would be the last time. There were frequent squalls and heavy showers, and the following north-easterly wind was unhelpfully strong and had a habit of repeatedly pushing *Bo* beam on in front of the wind. This was a time-consuming, frustrating and exhausting process to put right. Like most other problems, it crippled our speed. To counter these winds I deployed a small drogue, a mini version of the parachute anchor on the end of a thirty-metre line from the back of the boat. This would help prevent *Bo* from broaching.

For two days we carried on like this, making slow but steady progress towards the coastline of Molokai, the last island we'd pass before sighting Oahu. Despite Lane's passing, her legacy remained. Dark clouds loomed overhead and brought regular squalls, with strong winds and bursts of torrential rain. The waves, although diminished, remained formidable. The saving grace was both wind and sea were at least combined in pushing us towards our ultimate destination.

The really good news was that Sparky felt recovered enough from his injury to tentatively complete some short shifts at the oars. He was under strict instructions from me not to push himself too hard or too quickly, and more importantly not to break or lose any more oars. He'd already cemented his nickname, Sparky the Oar Slayer. It remained tough going but we were on track and the enormous threat of Lane had passed, leaving our goal in sight. It seemed we might finally be on the run home.

As we approached Molokai, I plotted a more diagonal course south as we traversed its long east-west coastline. I was planning on passing the western-most tip of the island, Ilio Point, little more than three miles offshore. That would give us the best chance of a good heading across the channel to Oahu. The drawback was the seabed becomes very shallow in that area, and there would almost certainly be very confused seas there after days of strong winds.

As we approached Ilio Point on 26 August, Chris's warning days earlier and my concerns were proved valid. The waves were nightmarish. They were large, flat and dangerously choppy with no discernible direction. We suddenly found ourselves in a stretch of ocean that behaved like the water sloshing around in a top-loading washing machine. It was impossible to row an accurate course and I decided attempting to maintain a safe distance away from land was our only concern. The wind, still blowing strongly from the north-east, would eventually push us west and past the island. All we needed to do was make sure we didn't get wrecked on its jagged coastline.

It was exhausting and soul-destroying work, and it took hours to finally pass clear of the island. I rowed as long as possible before

Sparky gave me a break and took over. It was really an exercise in keeping the boat upright and heading away from land until we broke free of the bizarre conditions the locals accurately refer to as 'Slop'. It seemed, no matter what, the Pacific Ocean was unwilling to give us any kind of easy run in.

Eventually and mercifully, we escaped the Slop and emerged into the slightly more consistent and predictable waters of the channel, finally clear of the western tip of Molokai. Right on cue the sun came out, and for the first time since Lane we had blue skies above us and relatively steady winds gently helping us towards the rapidly approaching finish line.

'This is how it must have been for the other two teams all the way in when they got here,' I said laughingly to Sparky.

The first and second placed teams had arrived in the islands long before us. *Danielle*, with the winning four-man team, had arrived on 26 July. The three girls on *Isabelle* made it in on 8 August, finishing second and creating a record as the first trio to race to Hawaii. We hoped they might still be in Hawaii for a shared drink, but doubted it. We were very much bringing up the rear.

As we progressed through day eighty-two of our voyage and what would hopefully be our last few hours on the Pacific Ocean, the idyllic conditions we initially experienced as we entered the channel began to change. The blue skies we'd so happily welcomed were replaced by huge banks of intimidating black clouds, the forerunners to violent squalls which swept in with bursts of gale-force winds, transforming the ocean around us. Less than twenty miles from the finish line we found ourselves once again battling formidable conditions which were threatening to destroy our voyage.

With the looming silhouette of Oahu punctuated by the lights of habitation on the island, we found ourselves in dangerously close proximity to land, with raging gales smashing into us. The only relief was that the squalls only lasted thirty or forty minutes, sometimes only ten or fifteen. As a result, the sea didn't have time to build too violently in response to their sudden impact. They did, however, make our life on board perilous. On the front of one of these squalls it was only a matter of minutes before we could be potentially courting disaster. There was no way I could ask Sparky to row in these conditions. As well as the risk of aggravating his injury, I was having to change direction repeatedly to keep *Bo* heading in a safe direction.

The squalls were violent and unpredictable mini-hurricanes. I eventually had to ask Sparky to go into the cabin as it was too dangerous for us both to be on deck together. We ran the risk of getting in each other's way if a sudden problem presented itself. He was reluctant to do that, simply because he felt he should be helping me. I could sense his frustration at the situation, but there was little he could do and it would take pressure off me to know he was safe in 'The Nest'.

I knew everyone at home or waiting for us on the island thought we were now completing the last few miles to the finish line without a care in the world. In reality, we were fighting a desperate, unexpected battle with the remnants of Hurricane Lane, which could render our voyage a failure at the very last moment.

I watched with a sick feeling in the pit of my stomach as the angry cloud formations of each squall formed in the night sky above me. The moon, which had been full the previous night, only added to the sinister and threatening atmosphere with its eerie light. A sudden temperature change would herald the arrival of the next squall, and in a matter of seconds winds in excess of forty or fifty knots would be smashing into the boat. Torrential rain and sea spray kicked up by the winds would make visibility almost impossible, and the boat would begin to heel and pitch violently in the suddenly confused sea.

Time and time again a violent gust forced *Bo*'s stern through the powerful winds, effectively pointing her on another heading, either away from the island back into the channel or much more dangerously in the opposite direction and directly towards Oahu's rugged coastline. Neither situation was good for us. The lulls between the terrifying squalls allowed at least a brief respite to recover. I was able to check the position and re-evaluate the course, even grab a quick drink of water.

It was an incredibly difficult balancing act. We had to approach the eastern coastline of Oahu as close as we safely could so as not to be too far east of Koko Head, the southernmost tip of Oahu on the eastern side of the island. The added fear was being too close to the coastline and being caught in one of the squalls and driven onto the rocks. Already I'd found myself on several occasions rowing away from the island for all I was worth to avoid disaster. In sailing terms, I was gybing down the coast, steering *Bo*'s stern through the following wind to pick the safest course to row to cope with the chaos generated by each passing squall.

By about 1 a.m. I realised I was becoming completely exhausted and desperate for just a short break. It was going to take several more hours of fighting through these squalls to make it safely round the southern headland and, quite honestly, I didn't think I was going to be able to do that without a rest. We were four miles off Oahu's eastern coastline, although in the darkness it seemed deceptively closer. I needed some sleep.

'Sparky!' I shouted.

He immediately opened the hatch and stuck his head out. I explained I needed him to spell me just for an hour so I could have a short break. He couldn't have been happier and emerged eagerly from the cabin to swap places. The conditions at the time were blustery but manageable and there was no immediate sign of another squall. It was as good an opportunity as I was going to get to safely take a break.

I set Sparky up at the rowing position and got him on the correct course. He could just about make out some of the clusters of lights on the island, which along with our newly extended 'shredded' Union flag flying above the cabin served as his reference point to steer. We were helped even more by the presence of the nearly full moon. I made sure he was OK and fully orientated then opened the hatch so I could crawl into the cabin.

'One thing, mate,' I said before I left.

'Yep?' he responded.

'Whatever you do, if I'm not out here again in an hour, wake me. Don't leave me a minute longer – you won't be doing me any favours, mate.'

'Why not?' he asked.

'Because if you keep rowing for much more than an hour, we'll hit land.'

After one of the most desperately needed sleeps I'd ever had on an ocean rowing boat, I woke to Sparky's loud calls from the deck. As I emerged into the cockpit, in the darkness Oahu stood menacingly over us, her silhouette even more defined as we closed in on her.

'What's that noise I hear?' Sparky asked as we swapped over.

I listened for a second and realised what he meant and smiled.

'That's the waves breaking on the rocks, mate. If we weren't quite so tied up, I'd suggest having that port now,' I joked.

'We're that close?' He asked.

'We're that close, mate,' I replied.

I swung the rudder over and began rowing a south-easterly course away from the breaking waves on the beach, mentally bracing myself for the next squall. I felt like a new person after my short sleep, reinvigorated and ready for the final battle to get in.

'Get some sleep, mate,' I said to Sparky. 'I'll wake you when we get around the point.'

He disappeared back into the cabin. 'Shout if you need anything,' he said, as he closed the hatch.

A few more squalls, mercifully shorter ones, smashed into *Bo* over the next few hours. I managed to keep on course for Koko Point despite their best efforts. It was as scary a time as I've ever had on an ocean rowing boat. There was so much at stake, so much riding on getting *Bo* into Waikiki and seeing Sparky step ashore to the hero's welcome he so richly deserved.

Each squall brought with it the threat of that being snatched away so close to the finish. I could see the lights of Koko Head in the near distance. The finish line was just six short miles along the more protected southern coast from there. All we had to do was round that point and we were as good as in.

I don't know if I was more exhausted emotionally or physically by that stage as I rowed through the last of the brutal gales generated by the squalls. I changed course frequently to ensure *Bo* remained close enough to round Koko Head successfully, but far enough away to not be smashed onto the rocky shoreline. After almost three thousand miles at sea our success would now hang on decisions regarding just a few hundred yards. I was terrified I was going to get it wrong in the darkness and let Sparky down at the last minute. I felt sick with worry.

Emerging battered from the latest duel with the seemingly endless series of squalls which had assaulted us, I realised I was looking at Koko Head from the south. My heart lifted. We'd made it. We'd finally rounded the headland during the chaos of the last squall and now with every stroke I took we were drawing further and further west within its protective shadow. The sea state was calmer, the wind had reduced and there was nothing but stars in the night sky as dawn approached.

It felt like I'd rowed onto a different ocean. The chaos and urgency of the previous twelve hours simply evaporated. It was as if it had never happened. I'm not ashamed to say I sat at the rowing position and wept with relief. I was in shock, I could barely take it in. We'd done it. We were going to make it.

There was still another six miles until the race finish line at the next headland, Diamond Head. It was an imaginary line drawn from the lighthouse out to a red navigational buoy just offshore. We'd anticipated crossing the finish line at 9 a.m. on 28 August. We were now several hours ahead of schedule, and everyone on the island was still asleep. Even without me rowing, the winds were edging *Bo* closer towards the finish line every minute. For once there was no rush.

The sun was due to rise for the last time on our Pacific row at 6.14 a.m. local time. I thought I'd wait until then to wake Sparky. I rang home to let my long-suffering mother know we'd all but cracked it and that we'd be crossing the finishing line in the next few hours. She congratulated us, wished us both well and said not for the first time, 'This will be the last row, Michael. Won't it?'

'Yes, this will be the last row, Mum,' I assured her, again not for the first time.

Then I sat back completely relaxed, allowing the weight and responsibility of the whole project to finally drain away. Beside me I could see the island of Oahu coming to life as the approaching dawn slowly diluted the night sky.

The different-coloured lights popped on in the shop fronts and businesses on the coast road. Vehicles began to fill that road with the bustle of early morning activity. Even the shapes and colours of the buildings were beginning to emerge. It had been over eighty-two days since I'd seen anything other than ocean. I drank it all in, with the pressure which had dominated every part of our Pacific row finally lifted, a huge weight was removed. Sparky was going to become the first blind person to row the Pacific Ocean. Nobody could say we hadn't earned it.

'Sparky!' I shouted. 'Come outside and check out our last dawn on the Pacific, mate.'

CHAPTER 29

CROSSING THE LINE

Sparky emerged from the cabin as the sun extinguished what remained of the night. We shook hands on a job well done. We could both finally see land, so we poured out a couple of small tumblers of port from the hip flask Dave Bull had provided and raised a glass to Oahu. I took the opportunity of becoming the first person to congratulate Sparky on becoming the first visually impaired person to row the Pacific.

'I'll drink to that,' he said, and poured out two more tumblers of port.

To prevent us reaching the finish line ahead of our welcome party we deployed the parachute anchor one last time. Then we made a final cup of tea with the last vapours of our rationed gas supply. Sipping our tea, we reflected on our voyage. It had been an epic adventure, one neither of us could have predicted, and more challenging than I could ever have imagined – but now, having completed it, all the more valuable an experience for that.

Ashore in Hawaii, Nat and Nikki had woken to the news we'd arrived early and were waiting close to the finish line for the race organisers to come out and officially see us in.

It was still quite rough as we approached the finish line and as the sun rose the wind speed rose with it. On *Bo* it seemed like just another day at the office, but when I saw the motorboats with the welcome party heading towards us, I realised how large the waves still were. I could see two boats in the distance, the smaller of the two almost disappearing at times between the swell, its bow leaping over the waves and crashing into the troughs. Strangely, on *Bo* it seemed perfectly stable.

Nat was on the smaller of the two motorboats and positioned herself in front of the helm to help contain her mounting seasickness. She was the only one looking directly forwards as they approached. Everyone else was expecting to see us off their port bow. As a result she was the first one to spot us.

'I can see them!' she screamed. 'I can see them!'

On *Bo*, Sparky and I began pulling in the parachute anchor for the final time.

'You OK to row, mate?'

'You try and stop me,' he growled.

As the two motorboats approached, Sparky set himself up in the rowing position and I steered from the cockpit just in front of the cabin hatch. I could see people on board waving and cheering. As the boats got closer, I recognised Nat, her broad smile stretched right across her face and her long blonde hair blowing in the wind. She had a blue striped frock on and looked fabulous. If I had any doubts how close we'd grown during the build up to the row, as our unlikeliest of relationships had slowly and unexpectedly developed, they were dispelled in a moment. The emotion at seeing her again washed over me as fiercely as any of the waves we'd encountered on our voyage. She waved back frantically. Then she disappeared.

'I've seen Nat,' I said to Sparky. 'But she's disappeared now.'

This happened several times over the next few minutes as the boats approached. It was only when we stepped ashore later that I found out that between each bout of frantic waving Nat was retreating to a large container which had been designated for her use. In fairness it was a very rough sea.

As the boat circled, I caught sight of Nikki and told Sparky. The smile on his face became even broader and they shouted across at each other half understood messages as the gathering wind stole their words.

'We need to get across that finish line,' I said to Sparky.

The increasing wind and waves were trying to force us past the Red Channel marker buoy which marked the left-hand edge of the finish line. We were running the risk of being pushed the wrong side of it. Sparky took to the oars and rowed as hard as he was able. Steering from the cockpit, I managed to keep him on a heading that should see us safely cross the finish line inside the buoy.

Some eighty-two days, sixteen hours and fifty-four minutes after we pushed off from Monterey Bay in California, that is exactly what we did. We were third overall in the race, and first in the pairs class, but most importantly Sparky had become the first and only visually impaired person to row across the Pacific Ocean.

A foghorn blast from one of the motorboats marked the moment. I leaned forwards, offering my hand to Sparky on the rowing seat. He left me hanging. Once again, I'd forgotten my rowing partner couldn't see and it was a few seconds before I realised and said, 'Mate, my hand's out in front of you. I want to be the first person to shake your hand.'

He laughed and offered me his hand and we shook. We'd only gone and bloody done it!

Two hours later Sparky was still rowing. He wouldn't stop. Regardless of any painkillers, the adrenalin alone would have fuelled his efforts to reach Waikiki Yacht Club. I continued to steer. We also managed to dispose of the remaining port on board with a number of toasts along the way to the many people who'd helped us achieve our remarkable goal.

The entrance to the harbour was marked by a sea the colour of mud, runoff from the heavy rainfall Lane had deposited on the island. It created a steady flow out from the entrance and markedly slowed Sparky's progress over the last half mile. There was a bump as we entered the outer harbour.

'What was that?' Sparky shouted, alarmed.

'Nothing, mate,' I answered, slightly embarrassed. 'We've just run over a turtle.' It was the only thing heading into the harbour slower than us.

Eventually we reached the entrance to the Waikiki Yacht Club and turned left. There were uniformed figures saluting us all the way, seemingly from a variety of different countries. We'd later discover it was Kiwi and Aussie officers along with their US counterparts in the North Pacific Command. They'd taken the time to come down and welcome two ageing bootnecks to Oahu.

I could see a large group of people at the jetty ahead and music was blaring out from what was obviously the yacht club. What we didn't know though was that back home in The Coach, people were watching a live stream of our arrival. Many of the people who'd supported us sat in the pub cheering as we rowed in. Big Frank, Dave Bull, Dave Sutton, Darren and Hayley and a whole host of locals who'd got behind the project. I don't really remember too much about the approach to the yacht club and coming alongside, but I'm told that just as we were approaching the jetty, I said, 'Well, that was a lot trickier than I expected,' which is probably the understatement of the century.

I do remember stepping off *Bo* and falling into Nat's arms and hugging her and telling her I loved her. I thought how wonderful she smelled and worried how badly I did.

Sparky was helped off by Chris and Nikki. The adrenalin that had fuelled his row into the marina depleted, he slumped exhausted into Nikki's arms. There was an enormous cheer. Everyone on the jetty was applauding. It was a wonderful welcome. The first of many Hawaiian leis were placed around our necks and

Sparky led the way shakily to the banquet of fresh fruit which awaited us inside the yacht club.

Sparky had done it. He'd become the first visually impaired person to row the Pacific Ocean. Nobody would ever be able to surpass his achievement. It was a world first. I doubt under the same circumstances anyone else could have completed it. Steve Sparkes had once been an exceptional Royal Marine. Standing on the jetty at Waikiki Yacht Club having rowed almost three thousand miles across the Pacific Ocean blind, overcoming an almost endless series of setbacks, one thing was clear. Steve Sparkes was still an exceptional Royal Marine.

EPILOGUE

The warm and emotional welcome at the jetty was only a taste of things to come. After enjoying the banquet of fresh fruit inside the yacht club, we devoured two long-dreamed-of steaks. Even though the Ala Moana Hotel was just a few hundred metres away, they had thoughtfully provided transport for us to make the short journey. We needed it. Exhaustion was engulfing the pair of us and Sparky's injuries were resurfacing painfully in the aftermath of his adrenalin-fuelled row in.

Entering the hotel lobby, still dressed in our rowing shirts and shorts, we were greeted by a guard of honour formed by the hotel staff. They applauded and cheered us every shaky step of the way into the building. It was as wonderful an experience as it was a humbling one, and would prove typical of the hospitality we'd enjoy in Hawaii.

A shower and a short nap in our hotel rooms was followed by an evening of seemingly endless interviews with TV and radio from across the UK and all over North America. My old friend Becca, our wonderful publicist, had done an incredible job generating and maintaining media interest throughout our voyage. We could not have been in more demand.

The row may have finished, but our responsibilities had not. This was our chance to repay our sponsors and most importantly to champion our two charities, The Royal Marines Charity and Blind Veterans UK. Everyone wanted to know how Sparky had survived Hurricane Lane. Everyone wanted to speak to us. And no matter how tired we may have been we were more than happy to speak to them.

It was after midnight before we finished, even then having to reschedule a couple of final interviews for the following day as we found ourselves barely able to string two coherent words together. Sleep beckoned for the pair of us, a long and uninterrupted sleep between clean sheets on stationary beds. We'd earned it.

Our return to the UK a few days later was equally overwhelming. It ran from the standard-bearers of the Royal Marines Association City of London Branch greeting us at Heathrow Airport, along with a cheering entourage of sponsors and supporters, to the endless messages and calls of congratulations and good wishes we received. Alone on the boat with only each other's company for almost three months, we'd had no idea that our adventures had generated such incredible support and interest.

A whole host of invitations came our way to attend and speak at prestigious events in the weeks and months that followed our return, culminating in November with Sparky and me attending The Royal Marines Charity Dinner at the Guildhall in London. In a banquet room oozing history, filled with almost five hundred guests, we listened to the incredible achievements of The Royal Marines Charity in the previous year and learned of the work that would need to be done in the years to come. It was great to know that our small contribution was helping to support such a forward-thinking, proactive and modern charity. Ultimately the evening would raise over a million pounds for The Royal Marines Charity, an incredible sum.

Keith Breslauer, the CEO of Patron Capital, sponsored the evening as he does every year. He let me know in advance that he had a surprise gift in store for Sparky and swore me to secrecy. Eventually Keith called Sparky to the stage to present him with an OrCam, a state-of-the-art device that attaches to the armpiece on a set of glasses. Via an audio facility it reads to the wearer any print or text they're looking at. It lets Sparky read a newspaper, a book or a menu. It can even recognise faces. More importantly, as Sparky would gleefully tell me later, 'I can even read the labels on beer pumps, mate.'

The presentation of the OrCam was a gesture typical of Keith's generosity and the icing on the cake of a project that against all odds had become a massive success on every level. Despite the endless challenges we'd faced, not only had we reached Hawaii but, more importantly, we'd captured people's imaginations.

One text out of the hundreds we received congratulating us summed it up best for Sparky and me. It arrived on our satphone after we'd survived Hurricane Lane and were battling through the last few days of the row. It was anonymous and there was no way of knowing where it came from, but the words struck a chord with both of us. It read:

I teach a special needs class. When you guys set off, I encouraged the class to follow your adventure. They loved it and soon became addicted, tracking your every move, every single day of your voyage. All I can say is thanks, guys, you have made a difference.

That's all Sparky and I wanted to do, make a difference. That one simple message confirmed we'd done that.

If there was a disappointment on our return to the UK it was that our Cockleshell Endeavour brother Steve Grenham wasn't around. He'd moved house, leaving his South Coast birthplace of Brighton for a more relaxed, mortgage-free existence in the north of England.

The signature song of our row across the Pacific had become Roger Whitaker's classic 'Durham Town'. The haunting and emotional lyrics in that song lean heavily on the premise that everyone for one reason or another seemed to leave old Durham town. We found it amusing that, in our absence, Steve had chosen to do exactly the opposite. He and his lovely wife Aicha had gone to live in 'Durham town'.

Steve's recovery remains on track. He still kayaks, and both he and his wife thrive on the less stressful life the north of England affords them – although he still won't put brown sauce on his breakfast. Steve is currently looking at completing a counselling course so he can offer more expert help for other recovering veterans in the future. He's come a long way.

As I write this, Sparky and I have decided on at least one more adventure together. We will take part in the famous ninety-kilometre Swedish cross-country ski race, the Vasaloppet. An accomplished skier despite his visual impairment, Sparky sees this as the perfect opportunity to exact revenge on me for putting him through the trials of our Pacific row. I haven't skied since 1984. Sparky has already christened the project Sparky's Revenge. What could possibly go wrong?

For my part, I'm taking part in the Yukon 1000 race in July 2020, paddle-boarding with another former Royal Marine one thousand miles from Whitehorse, Canada, to Alaska along the Yukon River to raise money for The Royal Marines Charity.

I also plan to continue establishing the Cockleshell Endeavour as a permanent and expanding resource for recovering veterans. It will be based on the principles that have worked so well on all our previous adventures: water-based challenges and races that allow recovering vets to work with former and serving personnel to achieve their goals and help get them back on track.

We're also creating an online resource to help recovering vets practise yoga, and also creating partnerships with industry to provide employment gateways to allow veterans recovering from physical and mental health issues to rejoin the workforce. The expeditions and races are important, but there are many aspects to recovery and ongoing fitness and health and employment are key elements to that. Steve Grenham is still very much part of Cockleshell Endeavour, as is our old friend Riggs.

Since the Pacific row, a documentary of Sparky's story based around our adventures is currently being produced in the UK. Ultimately, our aim is to see Sparky's Pacific adventure on the big screen as a full-blown movie. That may prove a challenge too far, however, as I discovered immediately after the race that Sparky has blotted his copy book quite spectacularly with one of the greatest film makers of our times.

A while back, Sparky had been taking part in an annual charitable walk across Dartmoor in Devon. It was a team event which he'd completed on a number of occasions to raise money for Blind Veterans UK. Sparky and a small group of blind veterans and a sighted guide would spend the day hiking across rolling countryside. Lots of different charities entered teams and there were hundreds of participants.

Unfortunately, the sighted guide for Sparky's team arrived late, missing the safety brief. He was handed a map and details of the route just before the team set off and was assured that everything he needed to know was in there.

Halfway into the hike the group came across a brand-new barbed wire fence stretched across a junction on the path they were following. The sighted guide looked at his map and checked the information he'd been given.

'No worries, guys, it says to take the track running to the north from here,' he said, looking up from the map with his arm outstretched pointing at right angles to their original path.

One of the group, with at least enough vision to recognise his whereabouts, interrupted him. 'No, that's not right. We always go that way. I've done this walk every year for the past ten years and the route is always along this path and over that hill. I don't care if there's a fence across the path. That's the right way.'

The sighted guide, who was taking part in the walk for the first time, tried to argue the point, but the blind veteran was having none of it.

Reluctantly, the guide conceded and Sparky and the rest of his team clambered over the barbed-wire fence and continued their hike up the hill.

Halfway up the hill they should have worked out something was wrong, as the grass was up to their waists and it was obvious no other teams had come that way.

'The guy saying it was the right way was insistent, though' – Sparky chuckled – 'so on we went.'

At the summit of the hill one of the team noticed there were literally hundreds of what seemed to be horseboxes in the distance.

'Must be some kind of Gymkhana going on,' he said.

Walking a mile or two further on they summited another small hill and found another brand-new barbed-wire fence stretched across the path. Again, the sighted guide looked to his map and issued instructions for an alternative route only to be loudly reassured by the blind veteran who'd completed the walk numerous times before that they were on the right path and to, 'Keep going! I know the way.'

The group once again struggled through the barbed wire obstacle blocking their path before carrying on their way. As they did so, the guide noticed in the distance a man running towards them. He was dressed in a high-visibility jacket and waving his arms and shouting something.

It turned out that the group was hiking directly across the set of the Steven Spielberg movie *War Horse*. To make matters worse, Spielberg had been waiting all day for the perfect light to film the climatic cavalry charge of the movie. The director had hundreds of horses and riders ready and waiting, only to see a humbling group of blind veterans stagger into shot at precisely the wrong time.

'All we could hear was Steven Spielberg screaming and cursing over the security blokes VHF radio,' Sparky recalled.

'It gets worse, though,' Sparky added. 'There was a team behind us from another charity, obviously not bothering to read their map – they'd just followed us along the same path. They'd walked straight across the set too, but they were dressed as giant green emus. I reckon Steven Spielberg must have thought we were taking the piss.'

Please don't hold it against us, Mr Spielberg. After all, worse things happen at sea.

ACKNOWLEDGEMENTS

The adventures in this book would not have been possible without a huge amount of support from an enormous number of people. I'm only sorry I couldn't mention every individual and organisation's contribution during the telling of this story. Here, though, is my chance to say a heartfelt thanks from me and on behalf of the 'two Steves'. Of course, I still run the risk of missing people, mainly because there were so many of you, so I apologise in advance if I have failed to mention everyone who helped. Rest assured your support was massively appreciated whatever form or size it came in and it all helped towards the remarkable successes we've managed to achieve and hope to achieve in the future.

So, in no particular order, here goes:

Thanks to The Royal Marines Charity for your constant support of all things Cockleshell Endeavour. Little we've set out to do would have been possible without it. I hope the money and awareness we've raised on our adventures has gone some small way to repaying that support.

Thanks to Blind Veterans UK (formerly St Dunstan's) for your support of our Pacific row. Meeting the terrific staff and members of your great charity has been one of the unexpected benefits of the challenge. Keep up the fantastic work – it changes people's lives.

Thanks to my great friends Maurice and Ann Stevens, stalwart supporters of many of my ocean-rowing exploits and equally supportive of all the Cockleshell Endeavour projects that followed. Sadly, Maurice passed away while I was completing this book so I'll not get the chance to get his greatly valued opinion on my literary efforts, but I look forward to hearing Ann's. You're much-missed, mate; future adventures won't be the same without you.

The Coach House, Rottingdean. My fantastic local pub, centre of the community, the catalyst for the Pacific row with Sparky and supporter of all our Cockleshell Endeavour projects. Darren and Hayley, the best landlord and landlady on the south coast (obviously that title further north is taken by Mum), great staff and fantastic customers, and a pretty excellent chef too! A large percentage of the money we raised on the 2018 Pacific row for The Royal Marines Charity and Blind Veterans UK came directly from Darren and Hayley's efforts at The Coach. A massive thank you, guys.

While on the subject of The Coach House, there's a long list of supporters from their loyal clientele, so here goes: thanks Little Kev, hope we took your mind off West Ham's woes for a short while, mate. The infamous gang of three who were there at the start of the Pacific idea: Dave Bull (The Port Giver), Dave Sutton (Sutton Workboats) and Big Frank (MD of FC Media); good blokes and great friends. Thanks to Rick Payne and his family at the Wagon and Horses and Jeff Halls (MD of 20six), and big thanks to Andy Brown for his personal support and for the sponsorship provided by his employer, FDM Group. Thanks also to Matt Hyde from Brighton Tools and Fixings.

Thanks to Stewart Sharman from FDM Group for all your help and support, and also to FDM's film-making guru, Greg Hughes, for producing a fantastic promo for our Pacific row.

Thanks to Norman and Rachel at Sussex Signs, Peter and the team at Logo Sports. Steve Brand and Mike Clift at Seahaven

Maritime Academy (even throwing me and Sparky into the Solent in January wasn't too much trouble). And thanks to Dan Temple and the guys at Seago.

Huge thanks to Mal and Jill, great friends and constant supporters and champions of the Cockleshell Endeavour projects and the Pacific row in particular. Even to the point of welcoming us into Hawaii. Great memories, guys.

Big thanks to Dave Spellman and Denise Penn. You find out who your friends are when you're up against it. Dave, thanks for all your help at a grim time and being a great mate – don't ever surprise me again, though. Denise, thanks for the lifetime supply of teabags for the trip; I'm still drinking tea made with them as I write this. Next time I might put you in charge of the gas cannisters too!

Thanks to Luke Francis – you saved the day introducing me to Paul and Dragon, mate.

And, of course, to Dragon Coin and its cofounder, yet another former bootneck done good, Paul Moynan, our title sponsor for the Pacific row in 2018. You were a lifesaver, mate. Not sure how we'd have made it to California without your help.

Andy Rice (MD of Elite Fabrication and Welding), it wasn't just like old days with you helping to sort our stainless-steel rowing positions for *Bo* at the last minute and your 'wets of tea' are still top drawer. Fantastic to see your company going from strength to strength, mate.

Thanks to Steve Talbert, a great friend for forty years and one of the first people to back our efforts in the early days of the Cockleshell Endeavour. Here's to the next forty years, mate . . . I've always been an optimist.

Thanks to everyone in the Falklands who supported Steve Grenham, me and the team when we returned to paddle around East Falkland and showed us such warm hospitality. Particularly

Gary Clement, Pinky Floyd, Carol and Terrence Phillips (sorry about using a year's worth of internet in one night, guys), John and Michelle, and thanks to Steve and Sue Luxton for putting up a motley crew of aging former bootnecks looking for a roof over their heads at the end of our paddle.

Thanks to Fergie and the guys from the garrison too, especially for the welcome fry up. Your efforts went a long way to making our expedition possible.

Thanks, of course, to our great friends Ricky Strange and Marty Gear, our support team, not just in the Falklands but throughout many of the Cockleshell Endeavour projects. Blokes like you have made me the man I am today . . . so you've both got a lot to answer for.

And thanks to Falkland Islander Kev Browning, CEO of Global Tunnelling Experts, sponsors of all the Cockleshell Endeavour projects and kind provider (supposedly on a temporary basis) of the third member of the Pacific crew: 'Rocky' (the penguin), our Falkland Island rockhopper mascot. I am working on prising him away from Sparky and returning him to you, mate. Honest . . .

And, of course, thanks to my fabulous friend Rebecca Saunders, a relentlessly enthusiastic supporter every step of the way with all we've done. You provided fantastic media coverage of all our adventures, but you exceeded yourself with the impact of our Pacific adventure. It still doesn't make up for your failure to ever make the tea when we worked together all those years ago . . . But you're getting there.

To my friend Keith Breslauer (Patron Capital), it goes without saying we're in your debt on so many levels. You and your family and your team at Patron have been a constant source of positive and practical support and encouragement throughout all our adventures and continue to be so. I look forward to flying the Patron flag on many future adventures to help recovering veterans.

Special thanks to my former employer and friend Paul Orchard-Lisle, a constant and staunch supporter of all my projects for over two decades now. I look forward to the next steak lunch, which I think may well be my shout.

Thanks to Dave, MD of 4x4 Vehicle Hire West Sussex Ltd, for helping out with transporting *Bo* to and from Southampton docks – service above and beyond, mate, cheers.

Thanks especially to Nat's family for their support and for welcoming me into the family – Monday nights have never been more fun or filling. Particular thanks to Mr H. for providing such a great soundtrack to our row across the Pacific (the theme from *Titanic* apart).

To my long-suffering mum and the locals at The Cowbridge House Inn, Boston, always the spiritual home of my adventures. To Sam Pesterfield, one of my oldest and best friends and the first person to offer support for the Cockleshell Endeavour project right at the birth of the idea. We've both come a long way since Kitwood Boys, mate.

To Daryl and Sabine, it would have been difficult to go back to the Pacific with any other boat than *Bo* – thanks for helping to make that happen, guys. I hope we added another great chapter to *Bo*'s incredible story and I look forward to following the next one . . . from a nice, comfy armchair.

To Al Hardman, thanks for all the time and effort training us up for more than one of our adventures. For an ex-Para you seem very at home on the water, mate.

To Tony Grenham, Si Reed, Phil Booth and Rob Osbourne, for all your support, particularly forming the A-Team to help get us to Westminster Bridge. Nothing quite like a steak and kidney pie to raise morale at 2 a.m., Rob. Cheers, guys.

To Riggs, the definition of a gentleman and a great mate. It would all have ground to a halt before it started without your constant efforts and energy, mate. Here's to more adventures in the future.

Thanks to Rory and Amanda Copinger-Symes for a great welcome in Hawaii and terrific hospitality during our stay. Thanks to our wonderful American friends Harry and Debbie, great supporters of all the Cockleshell Endeavour projects. Great to see you on the boat when we arrived, Harry.

Special thanks to Michele Mendez, sales manager at the Ala Moana Hotel, and Jade Carter, director of sales with the Mantra Group, for hosting us during our stay in Hawaii. A wonderful hotel, with fabulous staff. The warmth of the welcome into the hotel foyer you and your team provided for us rounded off a truly great day in the best way possible. The perfect introduction to Hawaii.

To Sgt Maj Anthony Spadaro (USMC), the senior enlisted soldier in the US North Pacific Command, thank you for a memorable lunch with a fantastic burger and an even more spectacular view, all rounded off with some quite remarkable company. It was an honour.

And huge thanks to two quite remarkable women. Nikki and Nat, without your constant support, love and backing, Sparky and I would never have made California let alone Hawaii. There's an ocean-rowing cliché that states it's always harder for those at home – although now you've had a chance to read the story you might think this row was the exception that proves the rule.

And, of course, the most important people to thank: Mr Grenham and Mr Sparkes. There would have been no story without the two Steves. Two blokes I'm lucky enough to be able to call friends, which is hopefully still the case after they've read this book. It was a privilege to be able to share these adventures with you both – I hope I've done you and your remarkable stories justice. Until the next adventure!

Last but most certainly not least, thank you for taking the time to read this story. I hope you've enjoyed it.

Mick Dawson

In memory of Allen 'Wayne' Lackey
19 April 1949 – 12 December 2019
A great man and a great mate who will be sadly missed.

THE COCKLESHELL ENDEAVOUR

The Cockleshell Endeavour project continues. Its goals are to provide an ongoing and sustainable resource for recovering veterans dealing with either mental health or physical issues. It's based on the principles that hopefully are illuminated in this book. Working together in teams on races, expeditions and challenges with likeminded people to start the process of recovery and rehabilitation. Using the values and principles taught in the service to get back on track; putting the other person first and above all never leaving a man behind.

If you wish to sponsor or support or just follow the Cockleshell Endeavour project or any of the events it runs, please go to our website: www.cockleshellendeavour.com.

If you wish to donate towards The Royal Marines Charity (our designated charity), supporting their ongoing work in helping serving and former Royal Marines and their families, you can do so through the Cockleshell Endeavour website or directly through: www.theroyalmarinescharity.org.uk.

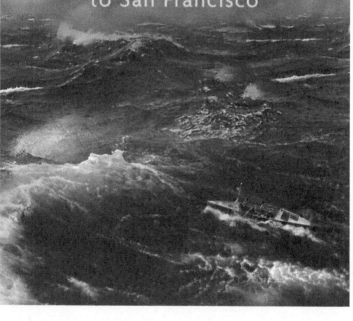

MICK DAWSON
ROWING THE PACIFIC

7,000 Miles from Japan to San Francisco

Rowing the Pacific: 7,000 Miles from Japan to San Francisco

On 8 May 2009 Mick Dawson and Chris Martin set off from Choshi in Japan to row 7,000 miles across the North Pacific to San Francisco . . . this is their story.

Crossing the North Pacific in an open rowing boat was one of the world's Last Great Firsts and, on his third attempt at this most challenging of all open-ocean rowing feats, Mick Dawson was determined to make it.

Storms, fatigue, equipment failure, intense hunger and lack of water are just a few of the challenges that he and fellow rower Chris Martin overcame during a back-breaking voyage of over six months. On 13 November, after 189 days, 10 hours and 55 minutes of rowing around the clock, facing the destruction of their small boat and near-certain death every mile of the way – they finally reached the iconic span of San Francisco's Golden Gate Bridge.

In this nail-biting true story of man versus nature, former Royal Marine commando Dawson takes on first the Atlantic and ultimately the North Pacific. His thrilling account of this epic adventure details how he and Chris propelled their fragile craft, stroke by stroke, for thousands of miles across some of the most dangerous expanses of ocean in the world, overcoming failure, personal tragedy and everything that nature could throw at them along the way.

Available now